2003/081

617.559
MCC

MISSING TEETH
A Guide to Treatment Options

02 DEC 2009
25 NOV
NOV 2010
NOV 2010
31/2011
OCT 2011
DEC 2011

Commissioning Editor: Michael Parkinson
Project Development Manager: Janice Urquhart
Project Manager: Frances Affleck
Designer: Erik Bigland

MISSING TEETH
A Guide to Treatment Options

J. Fraser McCord BDS DDS DRD FDS RCS(Ed) FDS RCS(Eng) CBiol MIBiol
Professor of Restorative Care of the Elderly,
University Dental Hospital of Manchester, Manchester, UK

Alan A. Grant DDSc MSc FRACDS FDS RCS(Eng)
Emeritus Professor of Restorative Dentistry, Queensland, Australia

Callum C. Youngson BDS DDSc DRD MRD FDS RCS(Ed) FDS RCS(Eng) FDS(Rest Dent)
Senior Lecturer in Restorative Dentistry,
Leeds Dental Institute, Leeds, UK

Roger M. Watson BDS MDS LDS FDS RCS(Eng)
Emeritus Professor of Prosthetic Dentistry,
Guy's, King's and St Thomas' Dental Institute, London, UK

David M. Davis BDS PhD LDS FDS RCS(Eng)
Senior Lecturer in Prosthetic Dentistry,
Guy's, King's and St Thomas' Dental Institute, London, UK

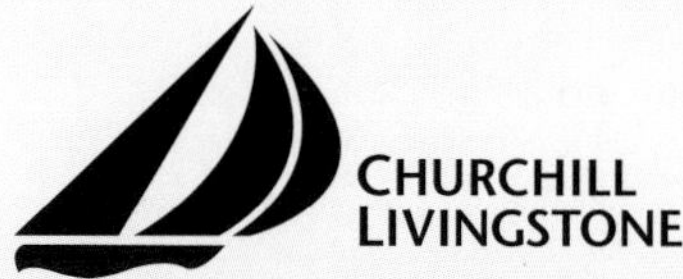

CHURCHILL
LIVINGSTONE

EDINBURGH LONDON NEW YORK PHILADELPHIA ST LOUIS SYDNEY TORONTO 2003

CHURCHILL LIVINGSTONE
An imprint of Elsevier Science Limited

© 2003, Elsevier Science Limited. All rights reserved.

The right of J. Fraser McCord, Alan A. Grant, Callum C. Youngson, Roger M. Watson and David M. Davis to be identified as authors of this work has been asserted by them in accordance with the Copyright, Designs and Patents Act 1988

No part of this publication may be reproduced, stored in a retrieval system, or transmitted in any form or by any means, electronic, mechanical, photocopying, recording or otherwise, without either the prior permission of the publishers (Permissions Manager, Elsevier Science Ltd, Robert Stevenson House, 1–3 Baxter's Place, Leith Walk, Edinburgh EH1 3AF), or a licence permitting restricted copying in the United Kingdom issued by the Copyright Licensing Agency, 90 Tottenham Court Road, London W1T 4LP.

First published 2003

ISBN 0 443 07153 5

British Library Cataloguing in Publication Data
A catalogue record for this book is available from the British Library

Library of Congress Cataloging in Publication Data
A catalog record for this book is available from the Library of Congress

Note
Medical knowledge is constantly changing. As new information becomes available, changes in treatment, procedures, equipment and the use of drugs become necessary. The authors and the publishers have taken care to ensure that the information given in this text is accurate and up to date. However, readers are strongly advised to confirm that the information, especially with regard to drug usage, complies with the latest legislation and standards of practice.

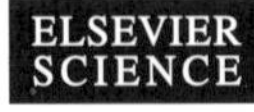

your source for books, journals and multimedia in the health sciences
www.elsevierhealth.com

The publisher's policy is to use **paper manufactured from sustainable forests**

Printed in China by RDC Group Limited

Preface

For centuries mankind has sought to replace lost or missing teeth; indeed, early 'practitioners of dentistry' used to ligate teeth removed from battleground corpses into the edentulous spaces of, presumably, eminent victors. There is also reference to a Mayan mandible which exhibited an implanted mollusc shell to replace a lost incisor. Removable prostheses were developed much later in the timescale of dentistry, and Pierre Fauchard, sometimes referred to as the father of dentistry, detailed removable prosthesis fabrication in his famous textbook of 1728. Many philosophies have been advocated over the centuries: indeed, there is no doubt that philosophies and treatment of missing teeth have evolved considerably over the last 50 years.

The decision to replace missing or extracted teeth may be made for a variety of reasons. The decision not to replace lost or missing teeth will in all probability be predominantly (but not exclusively), patient related. How to replace teeth becomes a subject of debate among the dental team, especially clinicians. Another area of potential difference relates to the design of a prosthesis, especially a removable one: although most clinicians may agree on whether a prosthesis should be fixed or removable, the nature of the design will often be subject to considerable variation. This is true of fixed or removable prostheses, but particularly so in the case of removable prostheses (RPDs). As Watt and MacGregor (1984) stated, this is because many features which are desirable in RPDs '*are mutually exclusive and the process of designing is a journey through a maze of compromises*'.

It is not difficult to understand why student clinicians struggle over the intricacies of treatment planning and of the design of a prosthesis, given their relative inexperience in the treatment of patients and the plethora of treatment philosophies and strategies that are advocated.

Most textbooks on the replacement of teeth tend to concentrate on either fixed or removable prosthodontic concepts and many admirable texts have been written. On the other hand, many excellent textbooks on the prosthodontic aspects of implantology tend to address practitioners with considerable clinical experience, and the treatment philosophies recommended might be unknown or poorly understood by less experienced practitioners.

The intention of this textbook is to serve as a clinical manual for senior undergraduate students and for graduate clinicians who are operating at a non-specialist level. Its purpose is to share our views on how to assimilate information, how to structure decision-making and, thereafter, in separate chapters, to deal with considerations for fixed, removable and implant-retained prostheses. As examples, 14 cases are presented in the Appendix, to enable the readers to follow design principles; we are sure that not everyone will agree with all aspects of the treatments carried out, but we are confident that the rationale of each case is robust.

We are also firmly of the view that the clinician should lead the dental team, and that this leadership should include responsibility for designing all prostheses appropriate to the needs of the patient; to do this, all of the areas in the chapters must be combined into a treatment plan appropriate for the needs (both current and future) of each patient.

J . F. McC.
A. A. G.
C. C. Y.
R. M. W.
D. M. D.
2002

Acknowledgements

This textbook developed as a result of discussions with delegates on courses and conferences at which treatment planning for missing teeth was a predominant feature. To the many delegates and students of prosthodontic dentistry who prompted us to look towards a textbook that addressed holistically the treatment of missing teeth, we offer our thanks. Similarly, we wish to thank Mike Parkinson and Janice Urquhart of Elsevier Science for their support and encouragement during the preparation of the manuscript.

Clearly we wish to express heartfelt thanks to our families for their encouragement and support, and to thank Anne, Janice, Anne, Kathryn and Morag for their encouragement which is, sadly, never fully acknowledged – we address that now. To many colleagues we offer sincere thanks for their words of advice and we wish particularly to acknowledge the assistance given by Trevor Coward, Harry Heyes, David Langley and Ray Richmond.

No textbook can be satisfactorily completed without a co-ordinating administrator and this project would not have been possible without the efficiency, support and thoroughness of Mrs Janet Lear, who also contributed to the text by improving the diagrams for the benefit of the reader, as well as acting as our best proofreader. To Janet, ably backed by Mrs Margaret Whatley, we all offer sincere thanks.

GWENT HEALTHCARE NHS TRUST
LIBRARY
ROYAL GWENT HOSPITAL
NEWPORT

Contents

1 Information gathering

INTRODUCTION

The loss or absence of a tooth or teeth may have a range of effects on the person concerned. For some people the effect of tooth loss may have severe social, professional or psychological ramifications. For others, tooth loss may be seen as a natural consequence of maturity. For example, 50 years ago in Britain, particularly in the northern part of the United Kingdom, it was not unusual for a man to leave school and be rendered edentulous prior to commencing employment in the mines or factories (Fish, 1942); for some younger women, prior to marriage, it was a norm at that time to have the maxillary teeth extracted and, as part of their dowry, to have these teeth replaced by a complete maxillary denture. Presumably the remaining teeth served as an innate fertility symbol, as they tended to be extracted after the birth of children, loss of calcium from these teeth being attributed to the effects of childbearing.

Fortunately, dental health education has produced significant benefits to the (dental) health of modern societies, and such philosophies are no longer encouraged. This fact, plus the widespread popularization of healthy teeth and gums and aesthetic smiles via the various media sources, has tended to make restorative dental treatment more sought-after. In addition, it is clear that the rise in demand has also engendered a rise in patient expectations, and this therefore places greater demand on the skills of the dental team.

For these reasons, it is essential that the clinician is able to diagnose the problem before deciding on how, or whether, to treat the patient. Socrates' daemon *'non primo nocere'* could well be translated in today's parlance as 'no diagnosis, no treatment'.

The purpose of this chapter is to provide the reader with a brief outline of some of the patient-related factors to consider before reaching the diagnosis. The next chapter will focus on decision making relevant to treatment planning.

There is arguably no 'correct' way to organize the information-gathering process, but with clinical governance in mind we offer the following systematic order as a reliable way to gather information.

Medical history

Whether the replacement or restoration of teeth actually benefits a patient from a purely medical perspective (excluding psychological or psychiatric perspectives) is debatable. What is incontestable, however, is that the restoration or replacement of teeth should never prove detrimental to the health

Health information

Health

1. Are you in good health?
2. Are you under the care of a doctor at the present time?
3. Have you ever had any serious illness or operation at any time?
4. Have you ever been in hospital, especially within the past year?

Illness

Do you suffer from, or have you had, any of the following:

Rheumatic fever?
Rheumatic heart disease?
Chorea (St Vitus dance)?
Congenital heart disease (blue baby)?
Heart murmur or valvular disease of the heart?
Anaemia?
Heart trouble, heart attack?
Stroke, paralysis or thrombosis?
Tuberculosis?
Bronchitis?
Chest pains?
Persistent cough or shortness of breath?
Fainting spells?
Blackouts?
Fits?
Fits or epilepsy?
Low blood pressure?
Asthma?
Hay fever (summer colds)?
Blocked nose
Eczema or hives (urticaria)?
Diabetes?
Jaundice (yellowing of the skin) especially after operation?
Arthritis (rheumatism)?
Kidney trouble?

Medicines

1. Are you taking, or have you taken, any of the following medicines, tablets or drugs during the past year? (a) Antibiotics (penicillin, etc); (b) tablets for high blood pressure; (c) nerve tablets for depression; (d) insulin or others for diabetes; (e) anticoagulants (to thin the blood); (f) cortisone (steroids); (g) tranquillizers (sedatives); (h) digitalis etc. for the heart.
2. Do you habitually take alcohol?

Bad reactions

1. Are you, or have you been allergic, sensitive or hypersensitive to any drug, medicine or anything else, such as: (a) local anaesthetic; (b) penicillin or other antibiotic; (c) sleeping pills; (d) aspirin or similar pain-killing drugs; (e) sticking plaster; (f) iodine; (g) any other drug; (h) any type of food; (i) ointments.

Dental complications

1. Have you been treated by the dentist during the past 6 months?
2. Have you needed treatment for bleeding following dental extractions, operation or injury?
3. Do you bruise easily?
4. Are you employed in any situation which regularly exposes you to X-rays or other ionizing radiation?
5. Have you had any bad reactions to any form of dental treatment?
6. Have you or your relatives had any bad reactions to a general anaesthetic (going to sleep for an operation)?

For women

Are you pregnant or taking the contraceptive pill?

For patients of African or Mediterranean descent

1. Have you or members of your close family suffered with sickle cell anaemia or Cooley's anaemia?
2. Have you had a blood test for these diseases?

Fig. 1.1 A useful form for recording the medical history of a patient.

of the patient. Equally, and with infection control in mind, the clinician should ensure that neither he/she nor any member of the dental team or other patients will be harmed as a result of providing dental care to a patient who is a carrier of an infectious disease.

For this reason, the clinician should follow a reliable algorithm to ensure that the patient's medical history is comprehensively recorded. Such an algorithm is illustrated in Figure 1.1.

Being armed with the known history, the clinician may, in conjunction with the patient's physician, determine the optimum way to plan the appropriate treatment.

For example, a patient with a history of rheumatic fever ought to be treated dentally in the most appropriate way to avoid the possibility of infective endocarditis (IE, and formerly abbreviated as SBE) arising. This may mean, for example, that therapy that is entirely supragingival may be rendered, as this will avoid trauma to the gingivae and soft tissues of the oral cavity; or it may mean that prophylactic antibacterial therapy is required where trauma to the soft tissues is anticipated or possible. Also, the medical history may reveal that the patient is taking anticoagulant therapy in the form of, for example, warfarin; this should alert the clinician to the potential for drug interaction with antifungal agents such as miconazole. Further examples are beyond the scope of this textbook, and these examples are given to demonstrate that the dental practitioner must be aware of the need to record the patient's medical history and drug therapy.

The dental practitioner should also be aware of the need to exercise clinical judgement and sound clinical observation at all times. It is likely that all clinicians will see a premalignant or malignant condition at least once in their working lives: it is to be hoped that these conditions will be recognized, or at least that their aberrance from normal will be recognized, and the patient(s) concerned referred appropriately. Obvious examples are squamous cell carcinoma and leukaemia. More obscure diseases may occasionally present, and such an example is seen in Figure 1.2. This patient wished to have his 'bite sorted out', as he could no longer bite his fingernails with his anterior teeth. He was a type II diabetic and was being treated for hypertension. He had no symptoms other than the fact that he had recently purchased three pairs of golf shoes in the last 3 years and each pair was larger than the previous pair. Clearly his dental problem was secondary to a medical problem, and a tentative diagnosis of acromegaly was made; he was referred to a consultant in oral medicine who confirmed the diagnosis. He was subsequently referred to a neurosurgeon for surgery on the pituitary gland, and his clinical case is included in the Appendix.

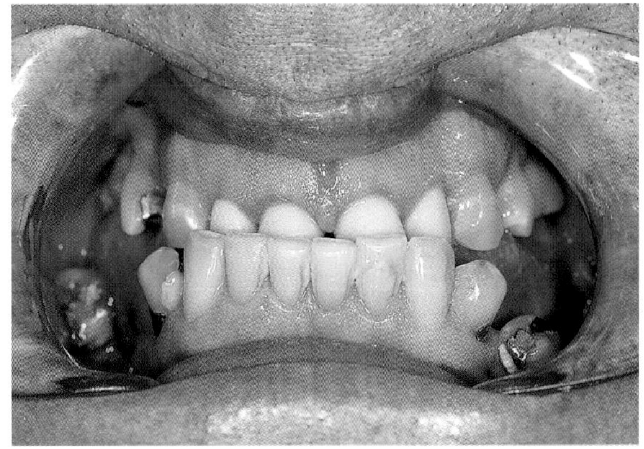

Fig. 1.2 This patient wanted his 'bite sorted out'. He claimed that he used to have a 'normal bite' but now had 'increasing difficulty in chewing efficiently'.

The need for the clinician to be aware of the potential for systemic factors to be mirrored intraorally should thus be self-evident.

Most dental clinicians receive instruction in, and are examined in, medicine and surgery as part of their undergraduate training. This is reflected in the membership diploma examinations in the UK Colleges.

Few older dental clinicians, however, have received training in the behavioural sciences and psychological and psychiatric medicine, although these aspects of care are now being introduced into the undergraduate curriculum. This is to be welcomed, as there is no doubt that there is a need to treat the whole patient, and the clinician who is not mindful of the behavioural basis of care may well find her/himself providing treatment that may not have an optimal outcome. Psychological profiling questionnaires such as the GHQ (Smith, 2001) have been shown to be of benefit in recognizing patients who are more psychologically problematic than the norm. Unfortunately, this adjunct is not in everyday use, although it is arguable that is should be used for many complete denture wearers who are being considered for dental implants (Smith, 2001).

The second area of patient history to be covered follows logically on from the first, and this is the area fundamental to dental treatment.

Dental history

Combined with the intraoral health status of each patient, this aspect of information gathering enables the dental practitioner to gain an impression of the patient's perceptions of dentistry and of their attitude to or motivation for dental care. It may also inform the practitioner on the dental care practised by the previous dental practitioner, and also of the patient's ongoing ability to maintain an acceptable standard of oral health.

Factors to bear in mind here are:

- The charting of the remaining teeth. In addition to obvious medicolegal aspects, this, in conjunction with the patient's wishes, may have a bearing on the treatment options.
- The status of the remaining teeth, i.e. are they intact, or have they been restored? If the latter, what is the status of the restoration and how long has (have) the restoration(s) been in place?
- What is the oral hygiene status, and is there periodontal disease present?
- Is there any prosthesis present? If so, is it fixed or removable? If the latter, how regularly is it worn and how has it affected the tissues adjacent to it?
- What is the status of the occlusion and is the patient able to function acceptably?
- What is the status of the masticatory apparatus? No assessment of occlusion should be performed without considering the posterior determinants of occlusion, namely the temporomandibular joints. Does the patient have any symptoms arising from the joints, e.g. is there limitation of opening, clicking or crepitus, or is there associated muscle tenderness?
- Does the patient have any soft tissue problems, such as bleeding, swelling or ulceration of the epithelial lining of the oral cavity?
- What is the reason for the absence of some or all teeth? Were any teeth ever present, or were they lost as part of orthodontic treatment, as a result of trauma, ablative surgery, or of periodontal disease or caries?

The medical and dental histories will reveal a considerable amount of information about each patient to the clinician. However, more information will be required, and this may be acquired partly by talking to the patient about their social habits.

Social history

It is essential that the clinician should elicit a comprehensive social history of the patient, and this may well involve questions about their drinking, eating and other social habits. For example, patients who drink alcohol excessively may suffer from gastric regurgitation, which can result in erosion of dental hard tissues. Equally, consumption of carbonated drinks may also result in erosion, and so prudence and caution are required in the way questions are phrased which will lead eventually to a diagnosis. Not all cases of erosion have an exogenous aetiology, and gastric reflux per se and an association with eating disorders may have to be considered.

Another aspect of social lifestyle is smoking. This has been shown to be detrimental to periodontal health and also to the process of osseointegration of dental implants, and patients who smoke must be made aware of these facts when treatment options are being discussed.

Other habits that should be investigated are perhaps more idiosyncratic and are associated with a combination of factors. Wear on the upper incisors (Figure 1.3a) and their proclination are attributable to a finger-sucking habit, but the effects of finger sucking are not wholly intraoral, as can be seen in Figure 1.3b. It is unlikely that dental treatment in isolation will be successful, and this perhaps illustrates the need to consider a broader approach to treatment after consultation with a behavioural scientist.

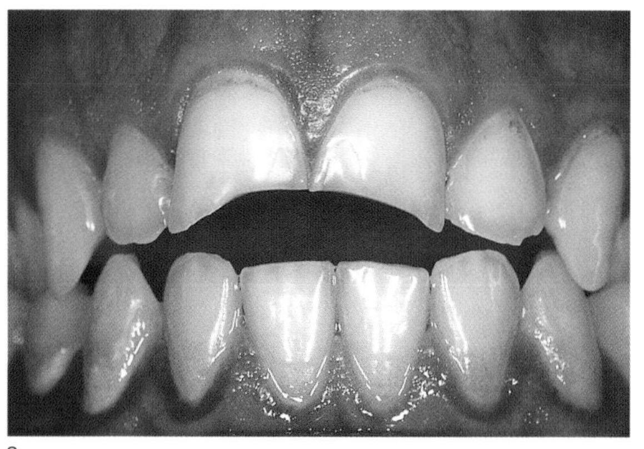
a

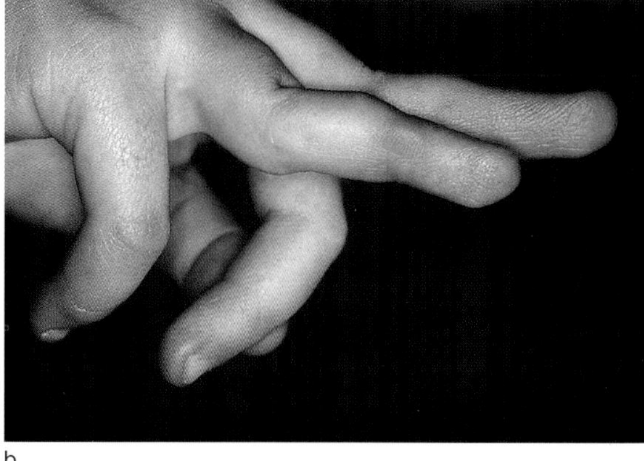
b

Fig. 1.3 (a) This young woman complained that her upper incisor teeth were becoming too prominent, 'like Bugs Bunny'; they also had an appearance suggesting that erosion was occurring or had occurred. (b) The same young lady had distorted fingers.

Other investigations

The above categories of patient-related investigations should provide a broad overview of each patient and will open the door for more specific investigations. Some of these are described below.

Vitality tests

It is essential to know the status of the remaining teeth, particularly those adjacent to edentulous areas and which may be considered as abutment teeth for fixed or removable prostheses. The vitality of these teeth may be determined via electric pulp-testing equipment, or by assessment of their response to hot or cold stimuli. These tests are not, however, infallible, as vital teeth may commonly give a negative response following trauma. For this reason, it is always prudent to combine these tests with a radiographic assessment (see below).

Periodontal assessments

In the same way that the health of the pulpal tissues of the remaining teeth should be assessed and recorded, so the status of the periodontal and gingival tissues should also be determined and recorded, not least for medicolegal reasons. A basic periodontal examination (BPE) will provide a broad overview of the periodontal health of all six sextants (where they are intact), and to this may be added plaque scores, pocket score charts and bleeding indices (Fig. 1.4). These measurements will be useful in the overall status of the patient but, as with the assessment(s) of the pulp, they should not be used in isolation but rather in conjunction with radiographic assessments.

Radiographic/imaging assessments

Although patients should not be exposed unnecessarily to ionizing radiation, there is a need to decide on the best available means of establishing the most appropriate imaging option (Whaites, 1996; National Radiological Protection Board,

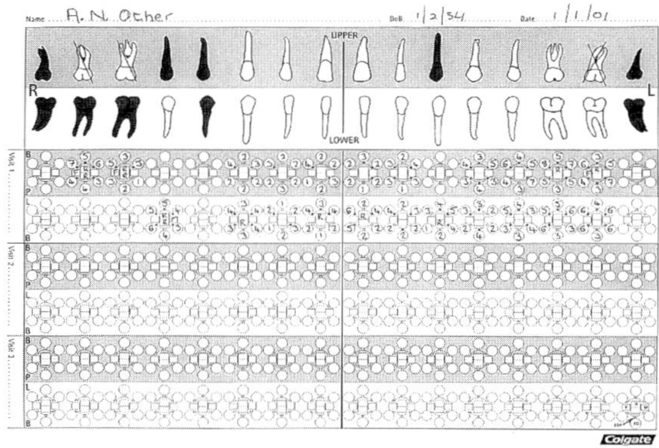

Fig. 1.4 A typical periodontal assessment form.

2001). Readers are referred to standard texts on dental radiology for details, but the clinician must be aware of the relative merits of periapical views, bitewing views and pantographic views as good screening and follow-up aids. Each has advantages and disadvantages and the clinician must select appropriately. Other imaging techniques are magnetic resonance and computed tomographic scanning; the former may be used to assess, for example, the soft tissues associated with the temporomandibular joints. The latter may be used to assess the edentulous ridges and associated anatomical structures with a view to implant placement, not to mention its usage in more extensive radiographic procedures, e.g. the assessment of the spread of malignant disease.

Ridge assessments

Ridges may be assessed according to form (Atwood, 1971; Moses, 1953), which is the cross-sectional shape of the ridge at the time of examination (Fig. 1.5a,b,c). This may indicate the potential for stability (a square-shaped ridge will offer greater support and stability potential than a wedge-shaped or a flat ridge), as the operator should assess the potential for the ridges to withstand displacement/compression. This may easily be performed with a gloved finger (McCord & Grant, 2000) to determine whether the patient experiences discomfort when the ridge is palpated digitally.

Ridge mapping may also be carried out to determine the form of the underlying bone and, by inference, the form and thickness of the mucosal tissues. Mapping may be carried out using the following technique:

- Record a minimally displacive impression of the ridge(s) concerned.
- Section the cast in the area concerned (Fig. 1.5a).
- Measure the thickness of the mucosa from the surface to the bone (after the appropriate placement of local anaesthetic) using a sterile probe with a rubber stopper (Fig. 1.5b).
- Scribe in the pattern from the stopper to the point of the probe and join up the outline (Fig. 1.5c).

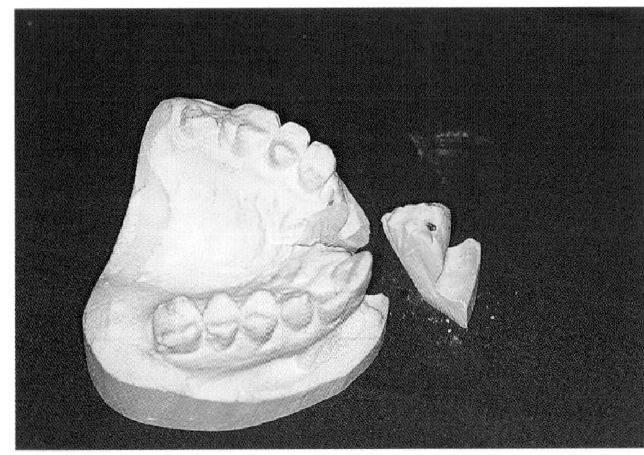

a

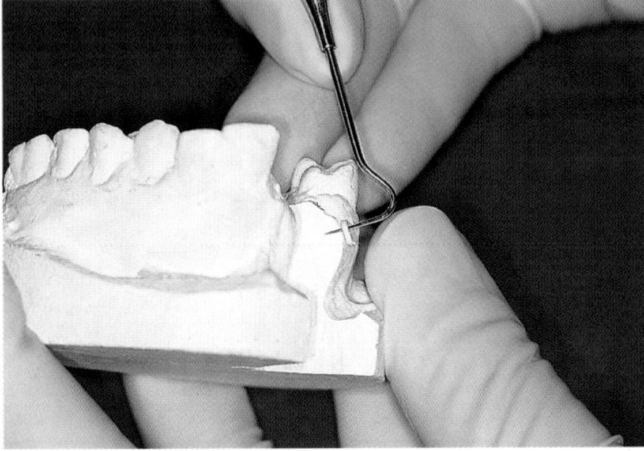

b

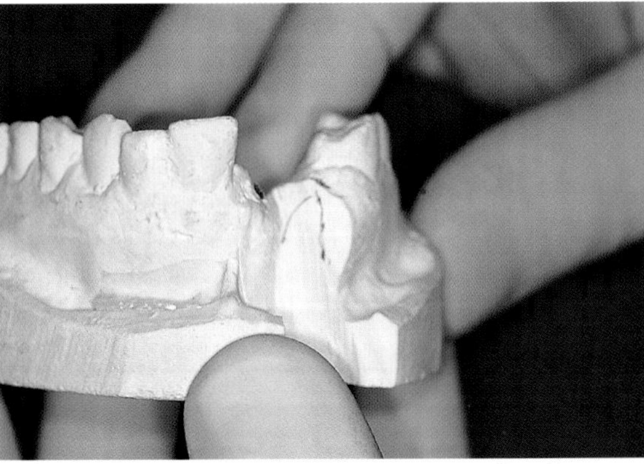

c

Fig. 1.5 (a) Section of a plaster cast of the edentulous area. (b) The probe, with the stopper in the appropriate place, is positioned on the cast and the depth of the soft tissue indicated on the cast. (c) A line linking the series of dots indicates the profile of the residual ridge.

(Alternatively, as was referred to above, this may be achieved radiographically via a CT scan, but this is much more expensive and is not readily available for most dentists.)

Bone assessments

Bone quantity and quality must be addressed and the former may be determined from the ridge assessment. Bone quality is usually assessed radiographically to determine relative densities. As there is a known association between osteoporosis and mandibular bone density, clinicians should be wary of the potential for further bone loss if osteoporotic bone is loaded unfavourably (Atwood, 2001; Devlin & Ferguson, 1990).

Tooth assessment

In addition to teeth being structurally sound they should also exhibit an absence of disease in the endodontic and periodontal complexes. There are other aspects of tooth form and position to consider. For example, the tooth may be malpositioned or over- or undererupted, and orthodontic therapy may be required to align the tooth more appropriately. Similarly, analysis of the tooth may indicate that its present restoration is sound but unaesthetic; for this reason, crowning or recrowning may influence the decision as to whether to make a prosthesis fixed or removable. More detailed assessment of the tooth may reveal that no undercuts are present and that the crown would require to be adjusted prior to the prescription of a removable prosthesis.

Monitoring

Assessment should not necessarily be considered as taking place on a single clinical visit. In cases such as tooth wear or non-cariogenic tooth surface loss, the aetiology may not be immediately apparent and, moreover, the data available from anamnestic use of diet sheets is often unreliable. Therefore, monitoring, either photographically and/or via study models, may be used to indicate whether the loss of dental hard tissues is ongoing or not (often the presence of staining may be an indicator that it is not). Similarly, soft tissue pathology may be monitored to determine whether resolution or progression is occurring.

Space assessments

When the dental arches or casts of the dental arches are being assessed, the clinician (and the technician) must consider the available space. Space, however, is three-dimensional, and therefore the use of study casts mounted on an appropriate articulator is to be recommended. The three dimensions to be assessed are:

1. *Horizontal space.* Here the clinician needs to determine whether the available space is sufficiently large to incorporate the appropriate amount of missing teeth (Fig. 1.6a,b). If it is too large the clinician may decide to accept the status quo, to reduce the space or, perhaps, to decoronate one of the abutment teeth to improve the appearance (Fig. 1.7a,b). Where the edentulous space is too small (Fig. 1.8a), again the operator (with the consent of the patient) may accept the status quo, elect to increase the space orthodontically (Fig. 1.8b), or decide to extract or decoronate one of the abutment teeth.
2. *Vertical space.* In this aspect, the clinician should consider interocclusal space and the vertical aspects of the abutment teeth. With regard to interocclusal space, the clinician ought to determine what space exists between the arches. For example, in edentulous areas lack of space (Fig. 1.9a) may require consideration of an increase in the occlusal vertical dimension (OVD) (if this is achievable without adverse reactions from the patient), preprosthetic surgery or, alternatively, acceptance of the status quo (Fig. 1.9b). Similarly, where the occlusion is maintained by teeth, the vertical overlap of the teeth and the room for, for example, a clasp assembly (Fig. 1.9c) or the pontic of a fixed unit (Fig. 1.9d) must be taken into account. There are several clinical options in all of these cases, but the important thing is to be aware of the presence of a potential problem.
3. *Coronal aspects of space.* This aspect of space consideration is particularly relevant to both removable partial dentures (RPDs) and

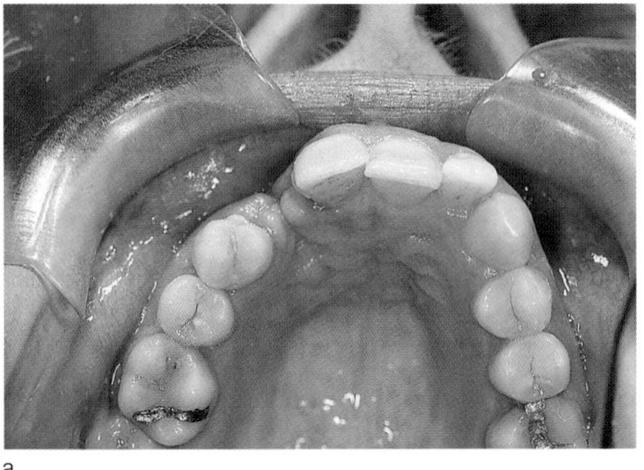

a

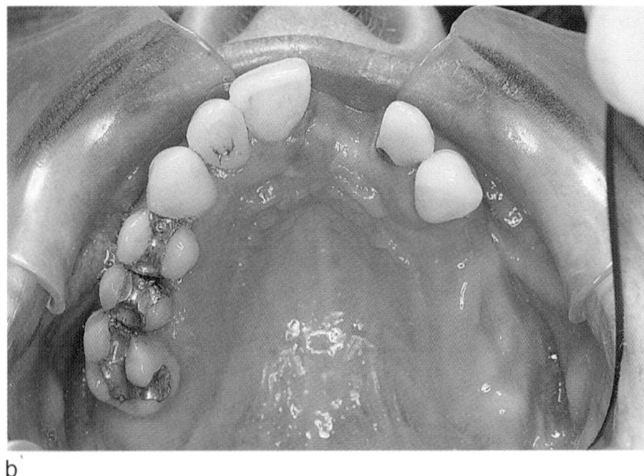

b

Fig. 1.6 (a) Here, two teeth are missing and, if one or both is/are to be replaced the clinician must determine whether they are to be supported by an implant or a tooth; if the latter, is the prosthesis to be fixed or removable? It is not considered good practice to restore such a gap in an otherwise healthy mouth with a mucosa-borne prosthesis. (b) Here there are several teeth missing and the clinician has to decide how many are to be replaced. Not all three molars need be replaced, and perhaps only one needs to be replaced with function in mind, although the patient may expect at least two molars.

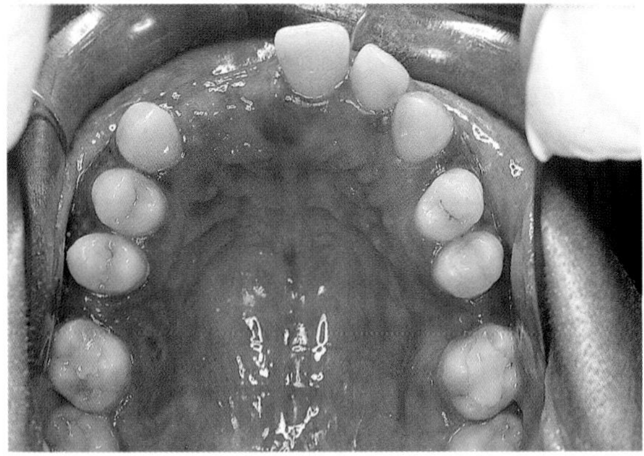

a

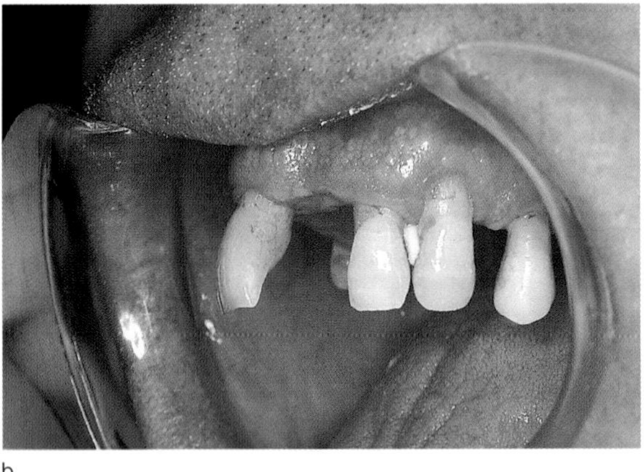

b

Fig. 1.7 (a) The anterior space was larger than the combined width of the lost teeth, but as the patient had spaces between her natural teeth no other treatment or no additional teeth were considered (see Appendix). (b) The single anterior tooth serves no useful purpose with regard to function, aesthetics or retention of the replacement denture. Consideration could be given to decoronating the tooth (after elective endodontics) and using the root as a means of supporting the denture.

implant therapy. Where mandibular premolar teeth particularly are lingually inclined, this will present a potential problem in the design of an RPD, and the space constraints may indicate two-part dentures or planned paths of insertion or tooth reduction philosophies.

The three-dimensional nature of the edentulous areas should be assessed during the aforementioned procedures, and this includes assessing casts of the patient's maxillary and mandibular arches on an appropriate articulator (see below). When this has been done, we advocate measured considera-

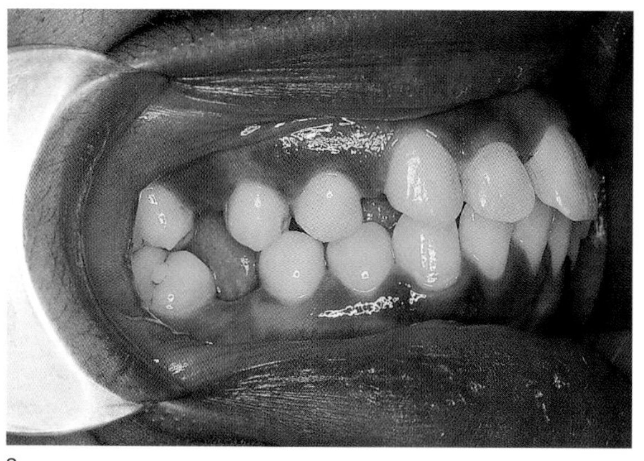
a

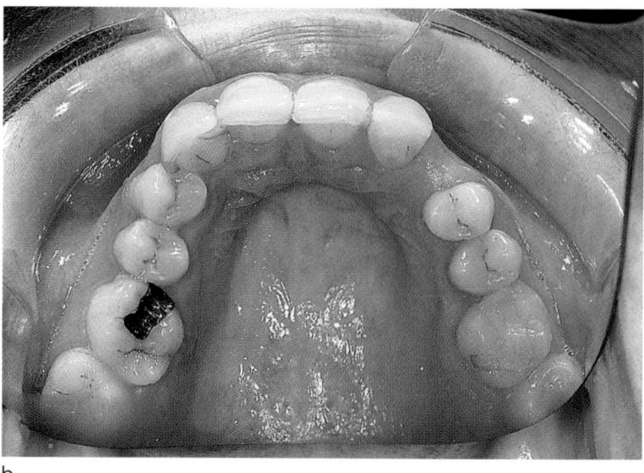
b

Fig. 1.8 (a) The space between the premolar and molar teeth is small; the size of the gap was accepted and a sanitary pontic planned in the denture. (b) The space for the canine is 4 mm less than the size of the contralateral canine; orthodontic treatment was carried out to increase the size of the space.

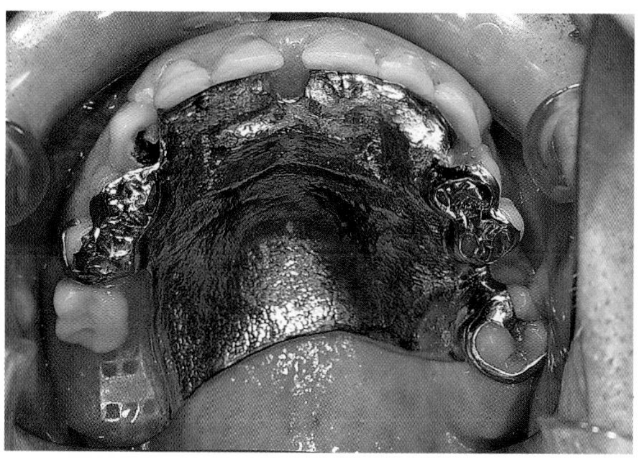
a

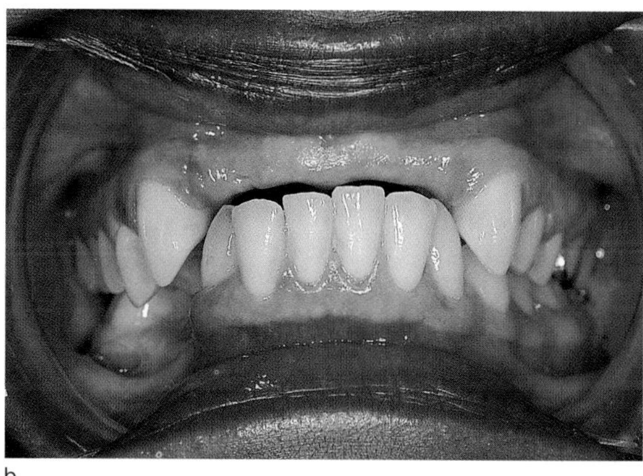
b

Fig. 1.9 (a) Lack of space in the vertical plane is overcome by an onlay denture, thereby creating space for the replacement saddle. (b) If teeth are to be inserted into this space, preprosthetic surgery is required to raise the teeth and supporting structures in the maxilla.

tion of all of the data accumulated, as outlined above.

This may not be possible after the first clinical visit, but it is only by thorough analysis of the information that a diagnosis may be made and, as was indicated above, diagnosis is essential before treatment strategies are offered. This naturally leads on to the next stage of the process, namely, what we do with the information? This is the subject of Chapter 2.

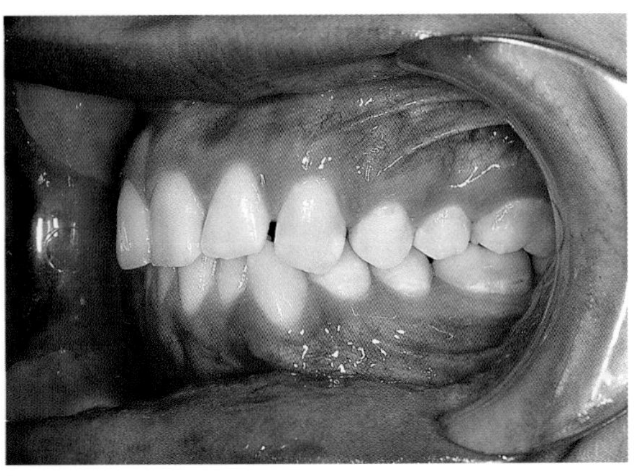
c

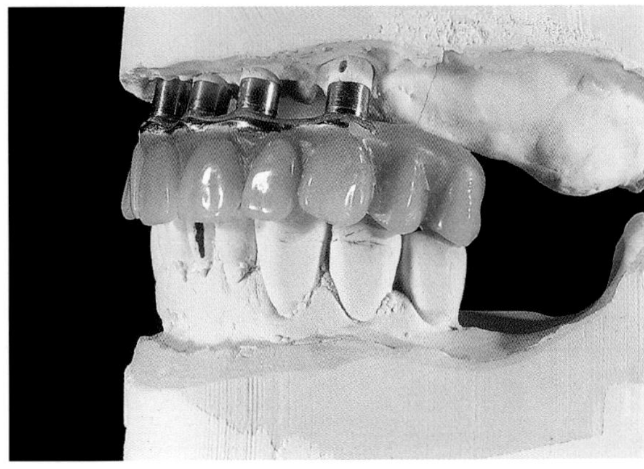
d

Fig. 1.9 (c) There is no space at present for a clasp assembly in this dental arrangement. (d) The pontics of this fixed–fixed bridge have assumed an idiosyncratic occlusal plane to accommodate to the opposing dentition.

REFERENCES

Atwood DA. Reduction of residual ridges. A major oral disease entity. J Prosthet Dent 1971; 26: 266–279

Atwood DA. Some clinical factors related to rate of resorption of residual ridges. J Prosthet Dent 2001; 86: 119–125

Devlin H, Ferguson MWJ. Alveolar ridge resorption and mandibular atrophy. A review of the role of local and systemic factors. Br Dent J 1990; 35: 29–32

Fish EW. The Englishman's teeth. Br Dent J 1942; 72: 129–138

McCord JF, Grant AA. A clinical guide to complete denture prosthetics. London BDJ Books, 2000

Moses CH. Physical considerations in impression making. J Prosthet Dent 1953; 3: 449–463.

National Radiological Protection Board. Guidance notes for dental practitioners on the safe use of X-ray equipment. London: Department of Health, 2001

Smith PW. Patients' perceptions of edentulousness. PhD thesis, University of Manchester, 2001

Whaites E. Essentials of dental radiography and radiology 2nd edn. Edinburgh: Churchill Livingstone, 1996

2 What we do with the information – decision making

INTRODUCTION

Most dentists will remember desperate moments in undergraduate clinics waiting to spy a patient whose dental complement or condition was such that they conformed to the needs of the requirements for 'sign-up'; in these circumstances, the hapless patients 'benefited' from the provision of either a removable partial denture (RPD) or a bridge, and the student equally benefited by satisfying the requirements for 'sign-up'. This might be seen as one reason for deciding on a treatment option, but it is not necessarily one that the clinician would care to repeat later on in his/her clinical career!

The factors that determine treatment selection are diverse (Kay & Nuttall, 1997). For example, we have all encountered patients who have essentially similar dentitions, yet we prescribe subtly different treatment options. Further, at certain times in our professional lives certain treatment philosophies prevail over others, and to render the scenario more complex we may not always demonstrate consistency in our decisions. Equally, two dentists may view the same patient and yet evolve dissimilar treatment plans.

The purpose of this chapter is not to look at why and how dentists select treatment options (for that, the readers are referred to Kay and Nuttall, 1997), but rather to assist the reader to form a template with which to begin to formulate a selection of possible treatment pathways. The principal clinical requirement is to select those options that are appropriate for the patient. It is necessary to present the possible range of pathways to the patient in order to obtain informed consent. The ultimate execution of the treatment involves many other considerations, and these will be discussed in detail below.

INTERPRETATION OF DATA

In Chapter 1, mention was made of the benefits to be gained from the practice of reflective thought when the data for each patient are considered (e.g. patient history, certain tests such as vitality tests, diet sheets etc.), examined and interpreted (e.g. radiographs) and assessed in detail (e.g. assessment of articulated casts), either in solitude or with a colleague or among colleagues. The benefit of this is that the basic parameters of dental assessment may be evaluated and measured against current guidelines or established practice. Although there are few real evidence-based guidelines in fixed and removable prosthodontics, the clinician ought to have an established practice on which to base his/her treatment plans. When the information

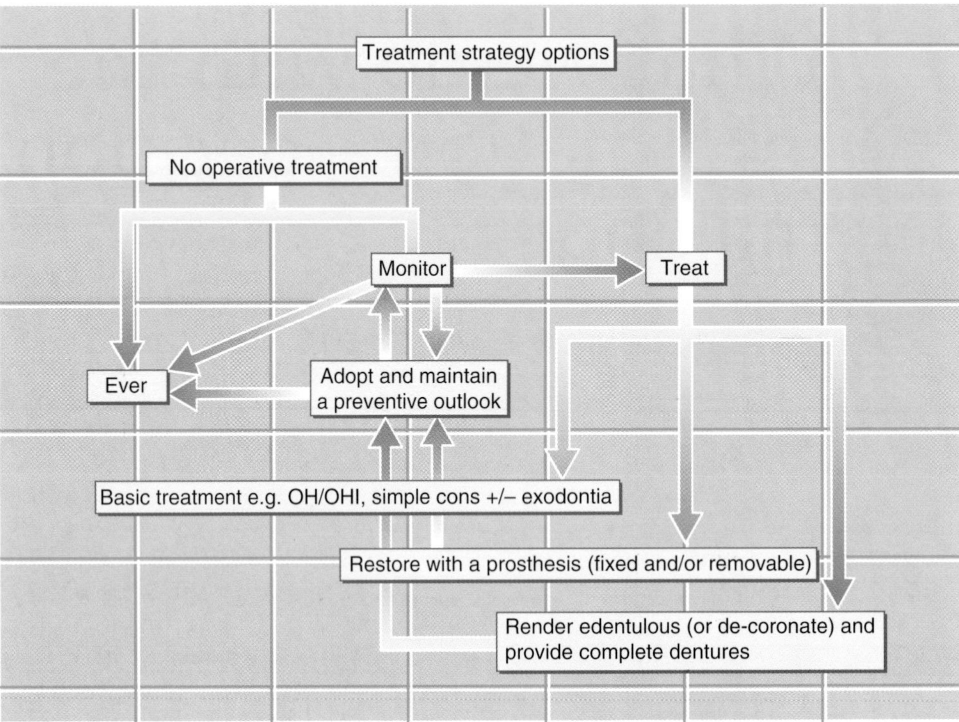

Fig. 2.1 A simple template which may be used to outline the first stages of treatment planning.

has been gathered, a simple empirical outline of treatment options is possible. This is illustrated in Figure 2.1, which requires that many other factors be considered before treatment strategies can be determined.

FACTORS INFLUENCING DECISIONS

As has been discussed, many factors have an influence on the formulation of the treatment plan. The first to be discussed will be those that relate directly to the patient.

Patient factors

A variety of factors may be relevant here, and although the list is not exhaustive the principal ones to consider, in addition to medical factors already alluded to, are age, oral hygiene, expectations of treatment and availability for treatment.

Age, for example, may be entirely relevant in the determination of the outcome. For example, evidence of wear in a young person may be an indication for treatment (assuming a diagnosis has been made), whereas it may not necessarily prompt treatment in an older patient – this is outlined in Figure 2.2; the presence of faceting here

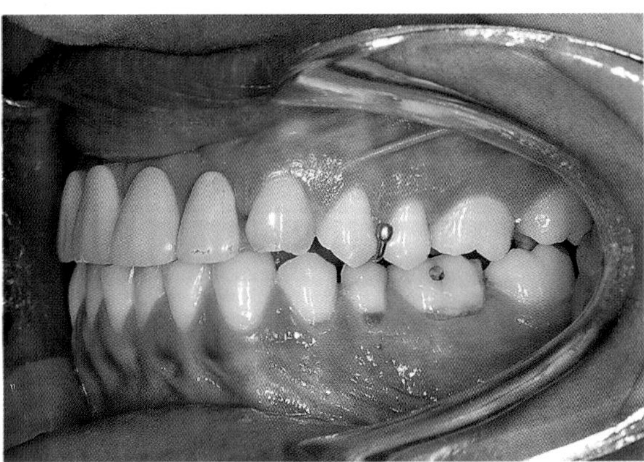

Fig. 2.2 Faceting on this canine will probably promote some form of treatment in a younger patient, but might not in an older patient.

might not cause concern in a patient aged 50 or more, but probably ought to in a 20-year-old.

Where orthodontic treatment is being considered to create/eliminate space, one should remember that the treatment may be quicker and the prognosis more favourable in younger patients: it may also be less socially compromising to prescribe fixed-appliance therapy for a younger patient. Another factor relevant to age is the relative size of pulp chambers in younger teeth; this may well determine the nature of crown preparation if such an option is required (see below).

From the BPE and basic examinations, the ability of a patient to achieve and maintain good oral hygiene should be determined. If this is problematic, elaborate treatment options should be delayed until such times as it is achieved. The alternative is to plan for transitional therapy if it is perceived that edentulousness is inevitable in the reasonably near future. In such cases perhaps a training denture should be considered to enable the patient to adjust to its use before being rendered edentulous (Fig. 2.3).

Coupled to this is the influence of social factors such as smoking, dietary habits etc. Reference has already been made to the potential for smoking to aggravate periodontal disease and to adversely affect osseointegration. It is the clinician's duty to explain this to the patient, essentially as a risk/benefit analysis.

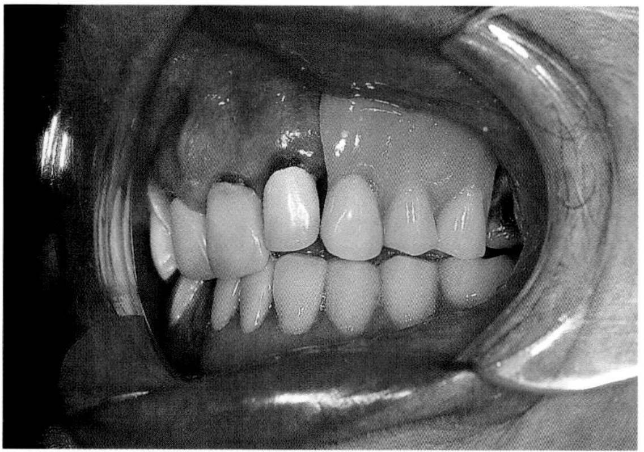

Fig. 2.3 This upper denture has been prescribed to enable the patient to – hopefully – become accustomed to and thereby facilitate the transition to a complete denture, whether conventional or an overdenture.

Two other factors that also have a bearing are patient expectations of treatment and ability to attend for treatment. In the former, it is essential that the clinician listens to what the patient wants. Failure to do so may result in the delivery of a treatment which is not what the patient wants. Equally problematic is the delivery of a treatment plan that a patient wishes for but which has no clinical sense: for example, a patient might request the extraction of all of his/her remaining teeth in the mistaken belief that such an action would solve all of his/her dental problems. The fallacy of such an expectation was highlighted by Applebaum (1984) when he described the expectations of complete denture wearers: 'A patient with a false eye cannot see, a patient with false legs cannot run, but many patients expect to look and function with dentures as well as, or better than, they did with their natural dentition'.

The need, therefore, to decide upon which treatment option to select needs a balance of knowledge and common sense. Coupled to this is the ability of a patient to attend. Pressures of work, either short term or long term, may influence the type of treatment provided, as may the health or medical condition of a patient, e.g. endodontic therapy in an expectant mother may justifiably be deferred until after the birth of the child and until the mother is able to attend for potentially lengthy treatments. Similar logistical problems are encountered over more elaborate restorative treatment in patients who may be living some distance from home while attending university, for example.

Clinical factors

The light-hearted scenario at the beginning of the chapter reflected, perhaps accurately, a not uncommon situation which ought not, however, to be reflected in the day-to-day practice of graduate dentistry, when it is expected that more meaningful decision making will occur.

Within the band of factors described as clinical are the clinician, the dental team and the suitability of the premises. The ability of a clinician to undertake a treatment option will be predicated by the amount of training and the experience of the dentist. A good example here is the use of precision attachments: it is not enough that the clinician provide precision attachments to retain and/or stabilize prostheses: he or she, in collaboration with the dental technician, should have included a plan for maintenance of the prosthesis(es) and the patient. Figure 2.4 outlines impression posts in extracoronal attachments as a means of replacing the male components in the denture; clearly, this means planning between the laboratory and the clinician and administrative efficiency in determining or recording which attachments are used, ordering the laboratory analogues and ordering the replacement parts. Alongside this is the need to have an additional (spare) denture while the definitive prosthesis is being upgraded. Similar examples abound where dental implants are concerned.

It is essential that the dental team works in an integrated manner, not solely for current treatment but for ongoing advice and maintenance. Another factor that clearly affects treatment options is the nature of the practice. The potential for outcomes in molar endodontics that satisfy current guidelines when operating microscopes and a range of obturating regimens are absent cannot be said to be great. Similarly, the potential for a stable outcome in a patient with an edentulous maxillary arch and a dentate mandibular arch (combination syndrome) is even more unlikely if a facebow transfer and intermaxillary relations are not transferred to an appropriate articulator (McCord & Grant, 2000).

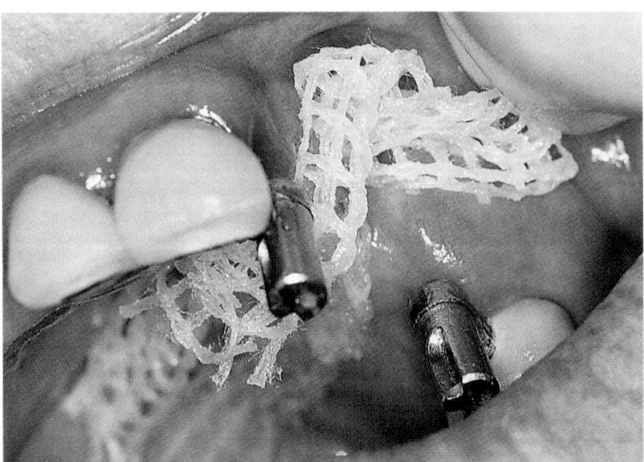

Fig. 2.4 Impression posts are placed in the female component of the extracoronal attachment prior to recording the impression for a replacement denture. This facilitates the technical process of fabricating the new casting.

On a more fundamental basis, in many dental surgeries access is via stairs: this may well present insurmountable barriers to some patients and therefore to certain treatments, as many aspects of restorative dentistry do not gladly lend themselves to domiciliary treatment (McCord & Wilson, 1994).

Patient–dentist relations

This factor undoubtedly has the potential to influence the course of treatment. The chances of a patient having the same expectations of the treatment as the dentist may not be high. Equally, the clinician should never assume that he/she has presented the clinical scenarios pertinent to each treatment option in a lucid, unambiguous way. Preston (1983) has outlined how dental jargon may easily confuse patients, e.g. words such as saddles, bridges and screw-in teeth have the potential to mislead. Coupled to this will be the personalities of the patient and the practitioner. It is inevitable that at some stage in a clinician's career there will be a clash of personalities: this ought to be recognized and highlights the need for a logical pattern to decision making.

Technical factors

Reference has already been made to all members of the dental team working optimally. Just as clinicians are advised against undertaking treatment of which they have little or no experience, the same applies to dental technicians and dental laboratories. Integrated planning is essential, and this will be highlighted in the case scenarios in the Appendix.

Other factors

The principal factor here is cost, either direct or indirect (e.g. time off work to attend). Many forms of restorative care, where lengthy assessment and treatment planning time is coupled to high laboratory costs, will result in expensive treatment and maintenance.

An empirical list of treatment options for missing teeth might include fixed and removable prosthodontics (including implant therapy), but for valid financial reasons, either short term or long term, the patient may opt for no treatment. Similarly, the cost of implant-retained complete dentures may prevent a patient having the optimal form of treatment, instead choosing either replacement conventional dentures or avoiding treatment altogether.

However, cost, as was stated earlier, is not necessarily directly related solely to treatment. Time away from work or from education may mean that a treatment option has to be deferred or another option pursued. Value for money is also a factor in cost, and if the treatment is tailored appropriately to the needs and expectations of the patient then it may well be perceived to have been 'worth it'.

A final consideration for cost is unrelated to finance: sadly, many patients have lost teeth, some totally, and the loss has been costly psychologically. The clinician must be aware that for such patients the replacement of teeth, especially by removable dentures, may not address the underlying problem. In such situations the need for liaison with an expert in behavioural sciences cannot be overemphasized.

In summary, the clinical and paraclinical factors to be considered when one is contemplating restoring an edentulous space are diverse, and include (McCord et al., 2002):

- Aesthetic factors
- Function
- Comfort
- Occlusal stability
- Speech
- Prevention
- Psychological factors.

When all of these have been considered in the light of all of each patient's details, then the decision making has to start formally. According to Anusavice (1992), decision making requires that a good clinician should:

- Reflect on the alternatives
- Become aware of the uncertainties
- Be able to modify his/her judgement on the basis of accumulated evidence
- Balance the judgement of the risks of various kinds
- Consider the possible consequences of each treatment option
- Synthesize all of the above in making a treatment decision.

In the course of day-to-day decision making the thought processes behind and associated with each clinical case are probably subconscious but, nevertheless, a process undoubtedly takes place, and human error can occur. The aggregation of data and decisions may be represented as shown in Figure 2.5.

A third perspective or dimension has then to be considered and that is a list of clinical options. These were illustrated diagrammatically in Figure 2.1. In brief, they may be listed as follows:

- No operative treatment. This is the simplest task and should reflect a healthy mouth and a healthy dentist–patient relationship. Supervised neglect could also be practised in this way, and this form of non-treatment is to be deprecated just as much as overtreatment.
- Monitor then act. This may be a typical format in toothwear cases, or where the clinician determines that the ability of the patient to achieve and maintain good oral hygiene requires assessment.
- Minor dental work with or without a prosthesis. This is perhaps the most common form of (restorative) treatment and will often involve simple restorations and perhaps periodontal and/or endodontic care or, on occasions, exodontia. Following basic care, a prosthesis (either fixed or removable) may be provided.
- Contrary to many teachings of the mid-to-late 20th century, not all missing teeth need to be replaced for masticatory reasons. Undoubtedly, patients who lose their molar teeth might perceive that their ability to eat will be impaired, but the convincing evidence of the research reported by Witter et al. (1990) has given an evidence base to the non-replacement of missing molar teeth. They called this the shortened dental arch concept, and it pertains

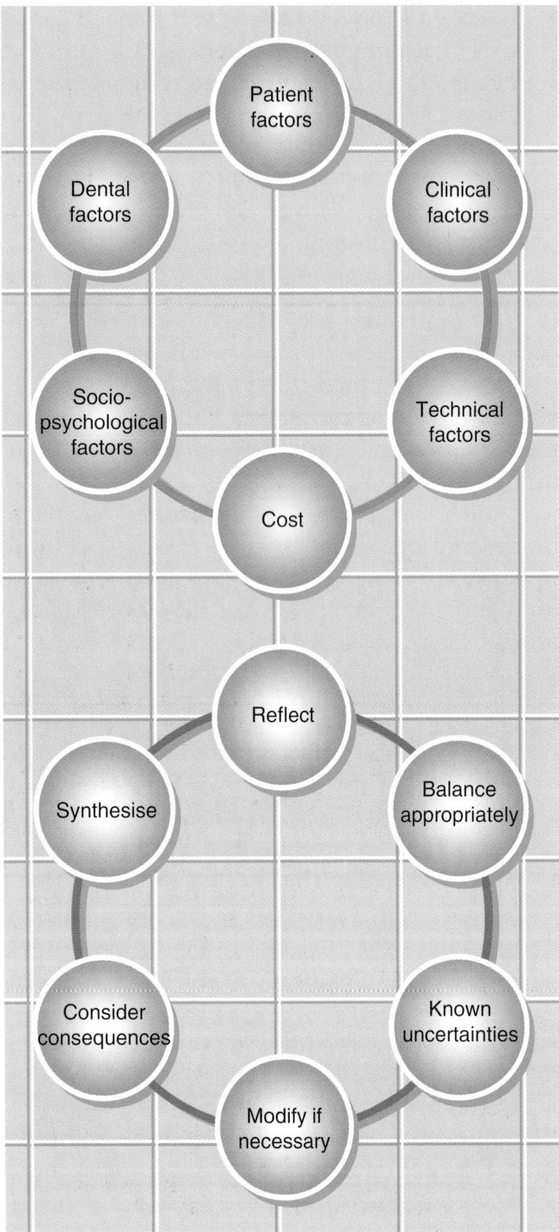

Fig. 2.5 The two 'wheels' of data and decision-making factors are presented on a ratchet-like arrangement. The potential for complexity of the process is thus apparent.

principally to the 45-year plus age group who have 10 healthy anterior units (teeth) in one arch opposed by 10 in the other arch. Given healthy teeth and periodontal support, the patients were judged to have satisfactory masticatory efficiency.

- As has been referred to earlier, however, sometimes the patient may wish to have the missing teeth restored for non-functional reasons (Glantz & Nilner, 1993; Hakestam et al., 1997), and here the clinician and the patient have to balance the risk of any prosthesis to the health/integrity of the remaining dental tissues against the perceived benefits (by the patient) of replacement of the missing teeth.
- Major work plus prosthesis. A range of procedures may be involved here and the cause of the extensive work required may be excessive toothwear, trauma, or congenitally missing teeth. A considerable amount of planning is typically required, with wax-up and trial dentures/splints being carefully assessed for form, function and appearance. In Chapter 1, for example, the need to assess space was highlighted, and the clinician may need to develop space for a restoration. This may be achieved via a removable splint (Fig. 2.6) or a fixed splint (Fig. 2.7) using the Dahl principle (Dahl & Krogstad, 1982) to create space for the definitive restoration. This will be illustrated in the Appendix, as will the preliminary planning stages of fixed and fixed and removable prostheses.
- As with the option above, removable prostheses may be immediate or definitive, simple or more advanced in design or, indeed, may also be an overdenture.
- The provision of dental implants. This will be discussed comprehensively in Chapter 5. In

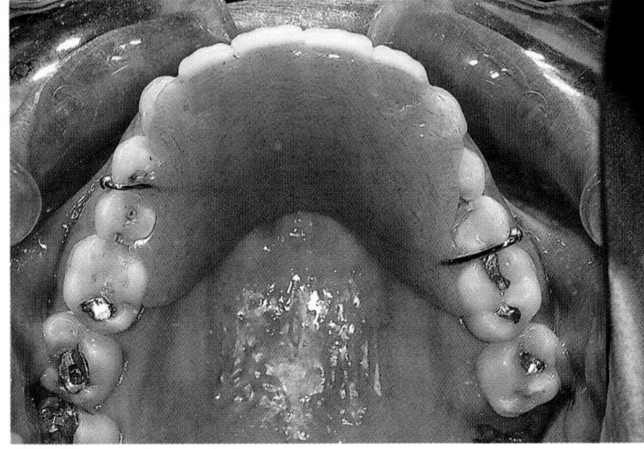

Fig. 2.6 A removable prosthesis which was prescribed to create space in the anterior aspect of the mouth.

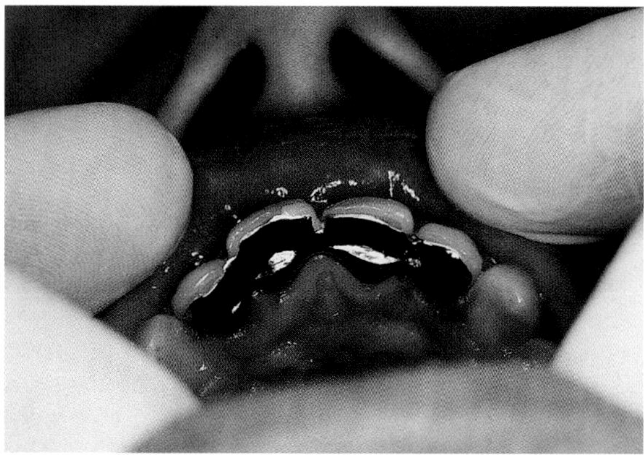

Fig. 2.7 A fixed prosthesis used to create space in the anterior aspect of the mouth.

this textbook, this category of treatment will include single-tooth implants restored by crowns, several implants restored with a fixed or a removable prosthesis, or an edentulous patient restored via an implant-retained and/or implant-supported prosthesis.

- As with the other aspects of prosthodontics, the need at all times to plan carefully is worth stressing both now and later.
- Consideration could also be given to the option of immediate or para-immediate replacement of a tooth with an implant body and the need to have an interim prosthesis.
- Render edentulous then treat. Unfortunately, there will be times when, for a variety of sound clinical reasons, rendering a patient edentulous is inevitable. The clinician has a responsibility to inform the patient of the consequences, both immediate and long term, of tooth loss and the changes in the residual ridges. The patient should also be informed of the likely lifespan of immediate dentures and of the need for replacements. With informed consent in mind, conventional wisdom would indicate that the possible usage of implants be discussed – albeit that other factors (e.g. clinical, cost, fear of surgery etc.) may preclude their use.

With the above range of possible treatment options the relevant areas should be presented to the patient so that informed consent may be obtained. When the treatment option has been decided on, the relevant planning may proceed in an appropriate manner. The relevant planning considerations for fixed, removable and implant-retained/supported prostheses will be discussed in the next three chapters. Each will attempt to render a process that is perceived by many experienced clinicians to be intuitive into one that is transparent to the relatively inexperienced. Although each chapter is intended to stand alone, none is intended to be considered in isolation: that would be in contrast to the philosophy of this book.

REFERENCES

Anusavice KJ. Decision analysis in restorative dentistry. J Dent Educ. 1992; 56: 812–822

Appelbaum M. Plans of occlusion. Dent Clin North Am 1984; 28: 273–276

Dahl BL, Krogstad O. The effect of a partial bite raising splint on the occlusal face height. An X-ray cephalometric study in human adults. Acta Odontol Scand 1982; 40: 17–24

Glantz P-O, Nilner K. Patient age and long-term survival of fixed prosthodontics. Gerodontology 1993; 10: 33–39

Hakestam U, Soderfeldt B, Ryden O, Glantz E, Glantz PO. Dimensions of satisfaction among prosthodontic patients. Eur J Prosthodont Rest Dent 1997; 5: 111–117

Kay E, Nuttall N. Clinical decision making. London: BDJ Books, 1997

McCord JF, Grant AA. A clinical guide to complete denture prosthetics. London: BDJ Books, 2001

McCord JF, Grey NJA, Winstanley RB. Planning partial dentures. Dental Update, 2001

McCord JF, Wilson MC. Social problems in geriatric dentistry – a review. Gerodontology 1994; 11: 63–66

Preston J. Communication, alienation, or confusion. J Prosthet Dent 1983; 48: 599–606

Witter DJ, Cramwinckel AB, van Rossum GM, Kayser A. Shortened dental arches and masticatory efficiency. J Dent 1990; 18: 185–189

3 Fixed prosthodontic options

INTRODUCTION

This chapter, in conjunction with Chapters 4 and 5, aims to render processes which are eventually intuitive into ones that are transparent and comprehensible to inexperienced clinicians.

In common with the aims of restorative dentistry in general (Ramfjord, 1974), the generic aims of fixed prosthodontics (fixed bridgework), as was stated in Chapter 1, are:

- To restore appropriate function
- To restore appropriate appearance (aesthetics)
- To provide comfort
- To provide stability
- A further prerequisite, however, is that the restoration should be maintainable by both patient and clinical professionals.

If a proposed prosthesis would not fulfil these requirements it should not be embarked upon, as there may be negligible benefit to the patient; indeed, there may be a potentially significant biological cost.

As has been alluded to in the preceding chapters, a guiding principle should be that minimally interventive procedures should be attempted in the first instance. To this end, resin-bonded bridgework should always be considered as a first line of therapy, although it may subsequently be rejected for patient-related or other reasons.

The majority of procedures practised in the United Kingdom at present are essentially replacement in nature, rather than de novo. This means, therefore, that for many clinicians the initial undergraduate and early postgraduation exposures to fixed prosthodontics will be of a conventional nature. For this reason, and because the factors that affect conventional bridgework also tend to affect resin-bonded bridgework, the former will be discussed first. It must be stressed, however, that no greater emphasis is placed on one form of bridgework than on another.

In the interests of clarity, and before proceeding further, some definitions will be offered to avoid confusion over terminology. Where possible, definitions for fixed and removable prosthodontics have been taken from the *Glossary of Prosthodontic Terms* (Academy of Prosthodontics, 1999).

A fixed prosthesis (fixed partial denture) is a prosthesis that is luted or otherwise securely retained to natural teeth, tooth roots and/or dental implants that furnish the primary support for the prosthesis. Fixed prostheses may be retained by conventional crown preparations (conventional bridges) or via composite-based resins to minimally prepared teeth where it is preferable that considerable enamel should be retained (resin-bonded bridgework). Occasionally fixed prostheses may comprise both conventional and resin-bonded components: these tend to be known as *hybrid* bridges.

For simplicity, the term bridge will be assumed to be synonymous with a fixed prosthesis (fixed partial denture) and will be used here as it is the one most widely used in the United Kingdom.

In common with other prosthetic solutions to the replacement of missing teeth, the bridge must be adequately supported and retained to withstand the functional forces to which it will be subjected, and the component parts of bridges are chosen to maximize this. Currently, nearly all bridgework is tooth (or implant) retained and supported, as described above. The principal exception to this is the spring cantilever bridge, which has a retainer remote from the saddle. However, this form of bridge is no longer popular. Abutment teeth must therefore be selected that are biologically capable of satisfying the aforementioned requirements.

COMPONENTS OF BRIDGES

Bridges have three 'components':

- A retaining element
- A connecting element
- An element which replaces the missing tooth/teeth.

In conventional bridgework the retainer is some form of crown cemented to an abutment tooth and incorporates a connector to the pontic (Fig. 3.1a).

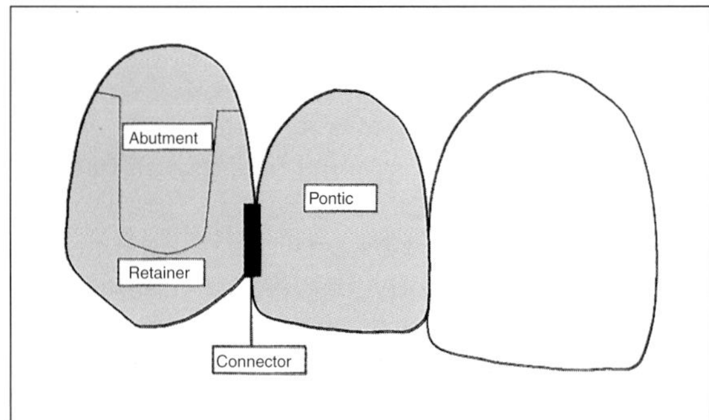

a

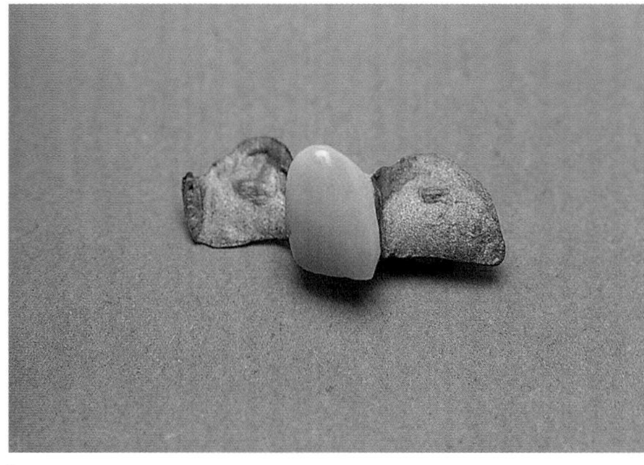

b

Fig. 3.1 (a) Example of a simple conventional bridge. The abutment on the retainer, connector and pontic are identified. (b) Example of a resin-retained bridge. Here the metal substructure comprises the wings and the infrastructure to the pontic.

In resin-bonded bridgework the pontic is connected to a metal wing that is cemented to an abutment tooth or teeth (Fig. 3.1b).

BASIC BRIDGE DESIGNS

Both conventional and resin-bonded bridgework may be of the following designs:

- Fixed–fixed bridges, where the pontic(s) is (are) retained by teeth on either side of the edentulous saddle (Fig. 3.2).

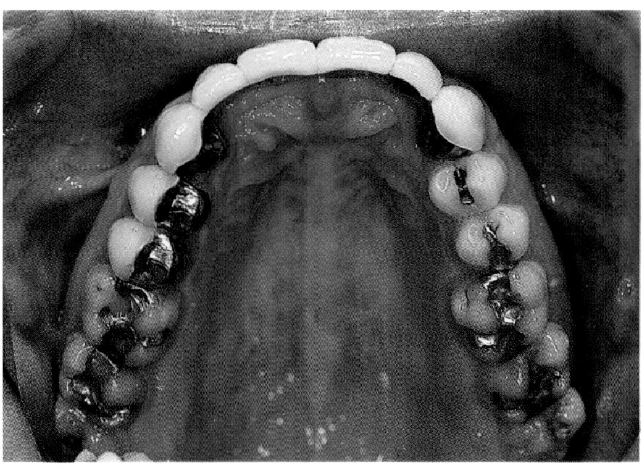

Fig. 3.2 Example of a fixed–fixed bridge.

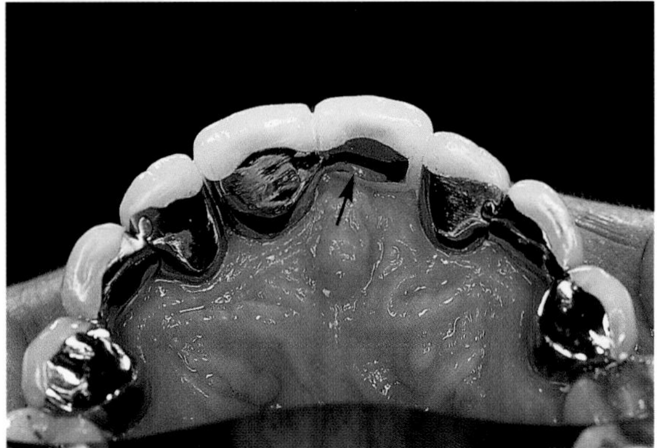

Fig. 3.3 Example of a cantilever bridge (arrowed).

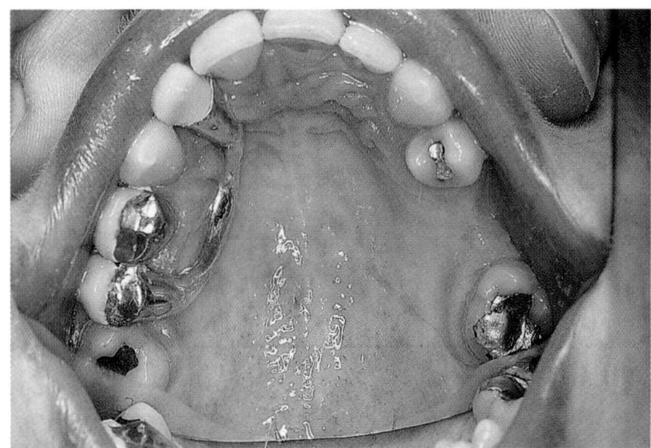

Fig. 3.5 Example of a spring cantilever bridge.

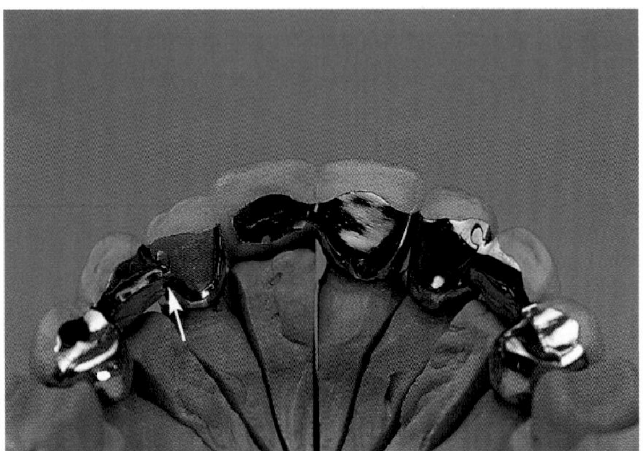

Fig. 3.4 Example of a fixed–movable bridge (arrowed).

- Cantilever bridges, where a pontic is retained by a tooth or teeth on only one side of the edentulous space (Fig. 3.3).
- Fixed–movable bridges can be fabricated where minimal movement, essentially vertical, can occur between the fixed and the movable components (Fig. 3.4). These are, however, mainly confined to conventional bridgework, owing to problems that may arise when used with entirely resin-bonded bridgework (see below). The movable joint is made up of a male component (the patrix) and a female component (the matrix). Convention dictates that the matrix should be placed on the distal portion of the minor retainer. This ensures that the **p**atrix is incorporated on the **p**ontic and the **m**atrix within the **m**inor retainer. The rationale for this is that the patrix will tend to be seated into the matrix (and will be subjected to compressive rather than tensile forces) during function, by virtue of the anterior component of force. There are many possible designs of patrix/matrix joints and the amount of support and 'stress-breaking' achieved will vary according to each design.
- Spring cantilever bridges. These are now seldom constructed. These bridges have a long connector from the retainer to the pontic (Fig. 3.5). This connector lies over soft tissue which, it is claimed, affords some measure of support for the pontic. However, the biomechanics of this design do not have a strong evidence base to support this assertion.

GENERAL INDICATIONS FOR BRIDGEWORK

The specific indications for replacing teeth by bridgework are similar to those for any prosthesis, and these were mentioned previously (see above).

The age of the patient is a factor in the success of bridgework, with an overall tendency to greater success rates for conventional bridgework in more mature patients (Roberts, 1970). In younger patients resin-bonded bridgework is often preferable, owing to the more conservative nature of the preparation of the abutment tooth/teeth, as well as the ability ultimately to resort to conventional bridgework should it fail repeatedly (Hussey & Linden, 1996).

Factors to consider

There are few systemic conditions that are direct contraindications to fixed prosthodontics that do not also apply to general operative dentistry. However, conditions that preclude a patient from sitting in the dental chair for long periods would suggest that other treatment modalities should be chosen. Without established periodontal, pulpal or periapical (periradicular) health, bridgework will fail or else iatrogenically aggravate existing disease. Occlusal or parafunctional forces must also be assessed to prevent trauma to the proposed abutments or the prosthesis.

The importance of the clinical examination, and the parameters to examine, was addressed in Chapters 1 and 2.

Particular clinical considerations

Periodontal considerations

All prostheses potentially aggravate plaque accumulation at the margins, owing to the presence of a restoration margin. For bridgework, active periodontal disease is a contraindication to treatment. The presence of gingivitis, although less problematic in affecting support, is also a contraindication. This is because of the difficulty in obtaining accurate impressions of the tooth preparation at the gingival margin, and the potential for the restoration margin to become visible following resolution of the gingival inflammation. No bridgework should be provided in the presence of poor plaque control or poor periodontal health, but it has been demonstrated that fixed bridgework can be successful in cases of successfully treated periodontal disease (Nyman & Lindhe, 1979) Figure 3.6.

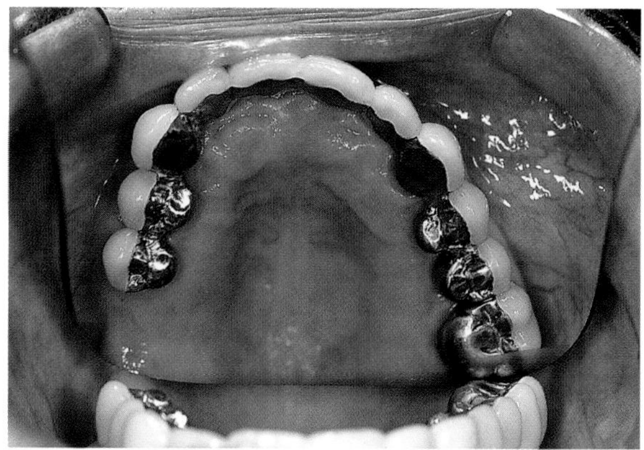

Fig. 3.6 Although the periodontal support available was much reduced, good attention to oral hygiene has resulted in a successful restoration of the dentition.

Pulpal considerations

The patient's caries risk should be assessed if there are a large number of restorations present. Bridge provision must be deferred until a stable situation is achieved and maintained.

Symptoms of pulpitis must be successfully treated prior to crown fabrication to ensure that the risk of pulpal pathology continuing under the bridge retainer is minimized. The removal of tooth tissue may result in a 'stressed pulp', leading to pulpal necrosis and probable periradicular disease (Saunders & Saunders, 1998). Access for root canal therapy then has to be gained through the bridge, usually necessitating a remake of the bridge.

N.B. An absence of pulpal symptoms is not necessarily a sign of a healthy vital pulp, and sensibility tests should be performed to confirm that a vital pulp is present.

Periradicular considerations

Teeth with untreated periradicular disease are unsuitable for use as bridge abutments for mechanical, ethical and medicolegal reasons. Where root canal treatment has been previously performed, the operator must ensure that it has been successful before commencing treatment.

The criteria for success include:

- Absence of pain, swelling or sinus formation
- Normal radiographic appearance or evidence of healing of periradicular pathology on sequential radiographs (European Society of Endodontology, 1994).

Previous endodontic treatment must be carefully assessed to determine whether the proposed treatment will compromise the endodontic result that is present. Where there is an obvious and simply remedied deficiency in the endodontic treatment/restoration, it should be revised prior to providing the bridge. The assessment of endodontic status, as was referred to earlier, relies on good-quality radiographic examination; periapical radiographs taken using film holders are therefore preferred.

Abutment core considerations

- *Vital teeth.* Any restoration within a proposed abutment tooth should be assessed critically, to determine whether the restoration is sound or if recurrent caries is present. If doubt exists then the restoration should be replaced, to establish a new core. Following the preparation of the tooth for this restoration, the clinician should determine whether there would be sufficient tooth tissue remaining to retain the core material. If this is in doubt, two options exist. The first is to replace the restoration with an adhesive material of acceptable strength, prior to preparing the abutment for the bridge. The second option is to prepare the tooth, with the expectation that the restoration will be lost, and then use an adhesive material to build up the core. The latter option is suggestive of less than ideal planning and is not our preference.
- *Endodontically treated teeth.* The processes involved in endodontic treatment (both during access to and preparation of the canals) inevitably involve the removal of significant amounts of dental tissue. Preparing the root for a post channel will result in an even weaker tooth, and the suggestion that conventional posts and cores will reinforce the root has been effectively disproved (Guzy & Nicholls, 1979). The effects of placing relatively new adhesive post systems on the strength of the remaining root, however, have not yet been determined by clinical trial.

  Conventional posts rely upon the post channel preparation, the close fit of a subsequent post and its morphology, and cementation for retention. The surface area of the post is inevitably less than for a crown preparation, and this can be considered a 'weak link' in fixed prosthodontics (see unmatched retainer). In addition, there is a significant risk of longitudinal root fracture if excessive occlusal forces are transmitted through the post.

  The use of a post is not a complete contraindication, however, and this option may be used (assuming the incorporation of a ferrule on to sound tooth and appropriate antirotation) in single-abutment cantilever bridges, where close attention is paid to minimizing occlusal loads. In posterior teeth, a conservative alternative to the placement of a post is via the Nayyar technique, (Nayyar et al., 1980), whereby the access cavity and a limited amount of the radicular preparation are used to retain a directly packed core material. The success of this technique, however, depends upon the selection of the core material and the amount of retaining coronal tissue.

Occlusal factors

As was mentioned in Chapter 1, preoperative study models should be obtained to examine the occlusal relationships and the relationship of antagonist teeth to the edentulous area. Where long span bridges are being considered, or where the patient's occlusal relationship cannot be easily determined, the study models should be mounted on a semiadjustable articulator using a facebow record and an appropriate interocclusal record (Fig. 3.7).

Factors related to the edentulous area

The length of the edentulous area is of considerable significance. Longer spans will be subjected

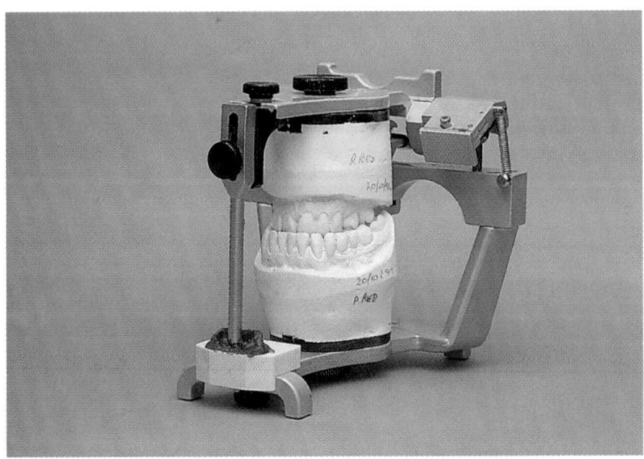

Fig. 3.7 The study casts have been mounted on an articulator via a registration in RCP.

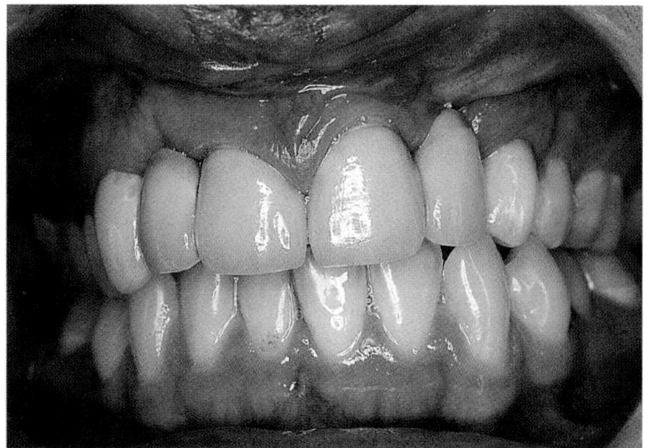

Fig. 3.8 The long incisogingival nature of the pontic results in a less than desirable appearance.

to increased compressive loads on occluding and laterally directed displacing forces when chewing. In the anterior part of the mouth, a further consideration is the curvature of the span. This is important, as greater leverage forces will be generated while incising on a very curved span, and these will transmit unfavourable forces to the luting cement and periodontium (Randow et al., 1986).

With regard to the form of the edentulous area, the degree of alveolar resorption can be critical in determining whether a fixed bridge is feasible. A problem that arises with gross alveolar resorption is the presence, gingivally, of wide embrasures that develop if normal tooth morphology is maintained. This may result in problems with speech or eating/drinking. The alternative of blocking the embrasures using long incisogingival connectors leads to a poor appearance (Fig. 3.8).

Factors relating to the teeth being considered as abutments

When selecting abutment teeth it is important to consider their position and orientation, as well as their coronal, root and pulpal morphologies.

The angulation of a potential abutment relative to the occlusal plane will influence its suitability, as axially directed forces on the abutments are required to maintain the biological integrity of the periodontium. A severely tilted bridge abutment will not exert forces axially upon loading. In addition, there may be problems in aligning retainers for fixed–fixed bridges without endangering the dental pulp (see below).

The retention afforded by the abutment is related to its coronal surface area (Potts et al., 1980) and therefore clinical crown height is of major significance. The relative size of the pulp space is also very important, as preparation for conventional bridgework could impinge upon this and compromise the abutment tooth's vitality. The material that will ultimately be used for the construction of the bridge will strongly influence the amount of tooth tissue to be removed. A compromise on aesthetics may have to be made to preserve pulpal vitality (e.g. use of gold, rather than porcelain bonded to metal crowns).

The root morphology of the abutment teeth may also affect the selection of an abutment, as longer, larger roots will better withstand the increased loading without exhibiting undue mobility as a consequence of adaptive changes. Anté's Law has been demonstrated to be without scientific basis (Nyman & Lindhe, 1979; Fayyad & Al-Rafee, 1997) but can be used as a simple guide to abutment selection.

Factors relating to retainers

- *Material selection.* For conventional bridgework there are currently two major types of retainer in common use. The first are constructed entirely from metal alloys (usually gold), whereas the second consist of porcelain bonded to metal. All-metal retainers are not generally considered to be aesthetic in the anterior region, although perceptions vary among ethnic groups. A relatively small proportion of bridges are constructed using all-ceramic materials.
  The retainers for resin-bonded bridgework will be discussed elsewhere in this chapter.
- *Retention.* This is a function of the surface area of the preparation as well as the amount of convergence of that preparation. In bridgework the preparation on the larger tooth therefore tends to be described as the 'major' retainer, whereas that on the smaller tooth is known as the 'minor' retainer (Academy of Prosthodontics, 1999).
- *Forms of retainer.* All-metal retainers may take the form of full veneer crowns, partial veneer

crowns (three-quarters or seven-eighths), onlays or inlays. However, the use of porcelain–metal full crowns, with their combined properties of aesthetics and strength, has largely superseded the use of partial veneer crowns as bridge retainers. The advantages of metal retainers relate mainly to the strength of material in thin section, as this obviates the need for substantial tooth reduction.

Full veneer crowns are structurally durable, totally enclose the tooth, and have the shortest restoration margin of those listed above. The preparation is usually relatively simple and, owing to its large surface area, is the most retentive form.

Partial veneer crowns are more conservative of tissue, as one wall of enamel (usually buccal) remains unprepared. However, as the preparation is less retentive and the resistance to displacement lingually is reduced, the placement of grooves is required. Even so, conventional partial veneer crowns demonstrate inferior retention to that of full veneer crowns (Potts et al., 1980). Furthermore, the lack of a complete cylindrical form to the crown means that it may flex under loading unless buccal offsets (upper retainers) or buccal shoulders (lower retainers) are incorporated into the preparation (Shillingburg et al., 1987). A longer restoration margin is present than with a full veneer crown, and this may increase the risk of recurrent caries.

Onlay restorations are less retentive and have a greater restoration margin length than partial veneer crowns, and should therefore be considered in only the most exceptional of circumstances. The same is true for inlays that suffer from a lack of occlusal coverage. It is possible that occlusion on to an abutment tooth might displace the tooth apically. However, if this forms part of a fixed–fixed bridge the inlay will not necessarily be loaded and the cement lute will fail around the inlay, with potentially catastrophic sequelae. The use of an inlay retainer may occasionally be acceptable as the minor retainer in a fixed–movable situation (see below) (Fig. 3.9).

Porcelain bonded to metal retainers are invariably full-coverage crowns and include some of the structural benefits of full veneer metal retainers. The disadvantage relates to the increased tooth reduction required on the facial aspect (1.1 mm minimum to 1.5 mm ideal) and carried into the proximal areas. This space is necessary to accommodate the metal coping and the overlying veneering porcelain adequately without overbuilding of the porcelain. If occlusal porcelain coverage is required this necessitates further occlusal reduction beyond that for metal, i.e. 1.5–2.5 mm compared to 0.5–1.5 mm (Shillingburg et al., 1987), which may adversely affect the height and hence the retention of the preparation.

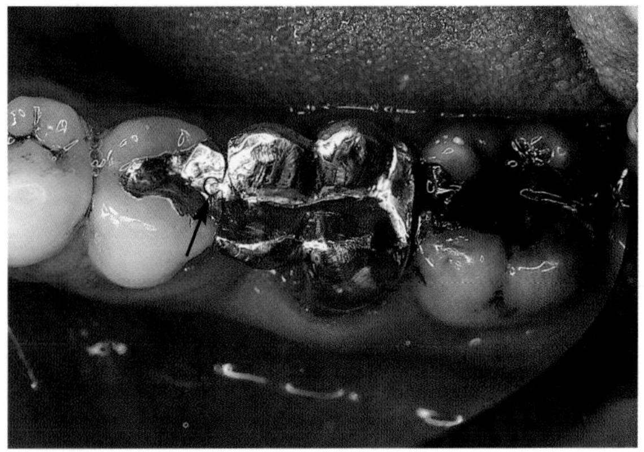

Fig. 3.9 The minor retainer is a gold inlay in this fixed–movable bridge (arrowed).

For all forms of retainer, the finishing line should extend 1–2 mm onto sound tooth structure beyond any core material present within the abutment to reduce the number and length of margins that may fail. This ferrule effect is considered to transmit more forces to the abutment tooth and protects the core–tooth interface from excessive forces (Sorrensen & Engleman, 1990). If the core extends subgingivally it is still important to finish on sound tooth tissue and, if necessary, limited soft tissue surgery should be performed to enable this.

Considerations relating to double abutting

Where it is judged that retention is less than ideal, a traditional approach is to increase the number of abutments in the bridge This will increase the surface area of tooth preparation and provide more support by involving more teeth. The

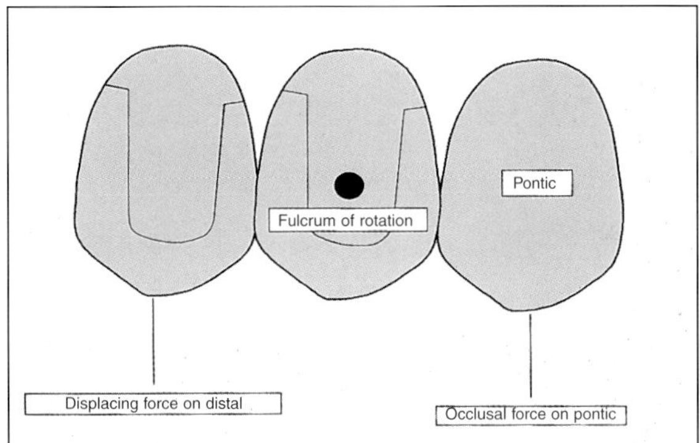

Fig. 3.10 This diagram indicates a problem associated with the distal abutment.

solution to a lack of retention may, however, cause a further set of problems. On occlusion on the pontic, the cement lute on the more distal abutment will be subjected to shear and tensile forces. As luting cements are not well able to resist these forces (Diaz-Arnold et al., 1999) there is a risk that the distal retainer will debond, but the bridge be retained by the more proximal retainer (Fig. 3.10). Double-abutted cantilever bridges have been demonstrated to fail mainly because of loss of retention and caries (Hämmerle et al., 2000), implying that the possibly increased retention and support is not highly effective.

Factors relating to matched or unmatched retainers

It is desirable that fixed–fixed bridges should have matched retainers (i.e. both retainers are full veneer crowns, or both partial veneer crowns, to avoid the situation where one retainer debonds but the bridge is held in place by the other). It is far better that if a bridge falls out it may be reassessed and possibly recemented, than that a partial failure goes unrecognized and gross caries occurs in the debonded abutment.

To overcome the problem of unmatched retainers it is possible to consider a fixed–movable design that allows slight movement between the pontic and the minor retainer. Benefits of this design include: a stress-relieving effect for the minor retainer, the same degree of support and axially directed forces provided by a fixed–fixed design, but less stringent parallelism between abutments. In some instances this 'stress-breaking' principle can be beneficially applied to longer spans and complex designs, such as those incorporating a pier abutment.

Stress breaking may help by reducing tensile/shear forces on a poorer retainer/abutment but still providing support. It should be recognized, however, that it has not been established how movable a joint must be to satisfy these requirements.

Technological factors related to design of the prosthesis

Difficulties can arise in the preparation, fabrication and service of a bridge cast in a single unit. Clinically, it is more difficult to achieve parallelism over a long span during preparation of the teeth. Furthermore, in the dental laboratory a long metal casting may distort during fabrication, or following porcelain application. Finally, there will be a tendency to flex during use (see Long-span bridgework).

Single cantilever bridges have the considerable biological advantage of requiring the preparation of fewer teeth. However, careful control of occlusal loading is paramount to prevent unwanted tooth movement. Previous suggestions that single cantilever bridges in the anterior maxilla were inadvisable (it was considered that rotation of the pontic might occur) have no scientific basis, although the need to plan the occlusal and soft tissue factors thoroughly should be self-evident.

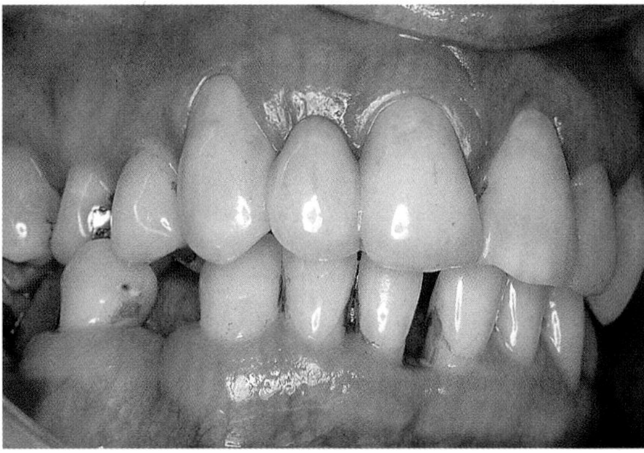

Fig. 3.11 The bulk required for the ceramic connector is evident here.

Factors relating to the connector

There is a fundamental requirement for the connector to be of sufficient magnitude to withstand occlusal forces exerted on the pontic(s) yet be of a dimension that allows the patient to clean the embrasure area below it using floss holders or 'bottle brushes'. Some all-ceramic bridges require a connector which is 4 mm^2 in area, and such a demand on size may, in many patients, compromise oral hygiene (Fig. 3.11).

Factors related to pontics

In addition to restoring aesthetics and appropriate occlusal contacts, these should provide minimal tissue contact. This is important to allow the patient to carry out effective plaque removal to prevent gingival inflammation under the pontic (Fig. 3.12).

Many types of pontic have been designed to overcome deficiencies in the available materials. As dental technology has improved, however, the range has diminished and there are only a few basic forms currently being used.

- *Modified ridge lap.* This is most often used in the maxillary anterior/premolar area and allows good function without compromising aesthetics (Fig. 3.13). There is a relatively large surface area of tissue contact, but the design allows simple cleaning. The presence of soft tis-

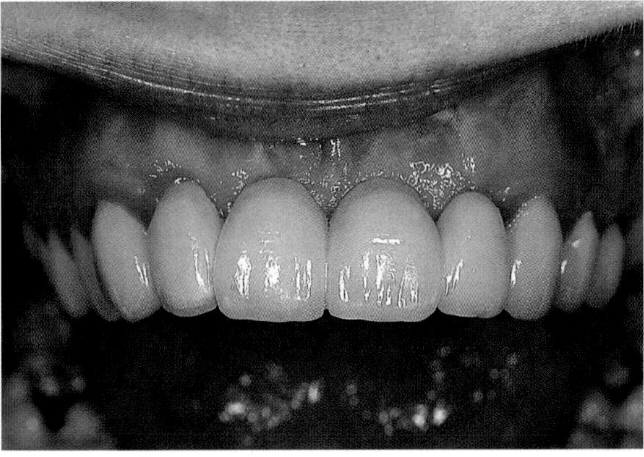

Fig. 3.13 The appearance of this bridge has not been compromised by this modified ridge-lap design.

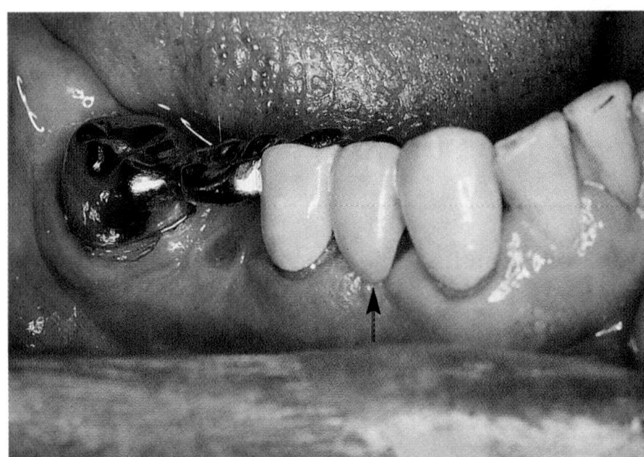

Fig. 3.14 Example of a bullet pontic (arrowed).

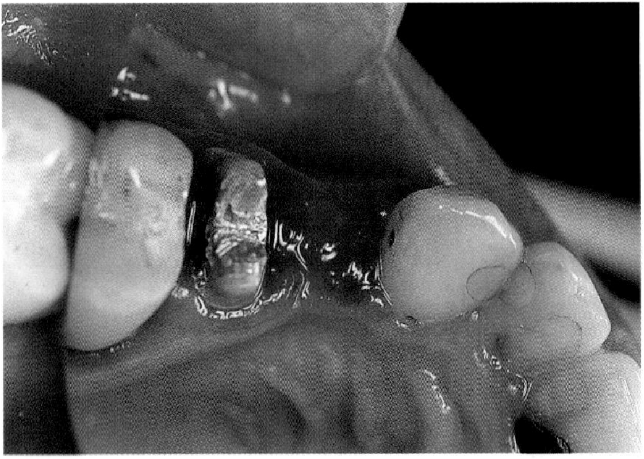

Fig. 3.12 Poor design of the pontic, in association with poor oral hygiene, has resulted in gingival inflammation under the (removed) bridge.

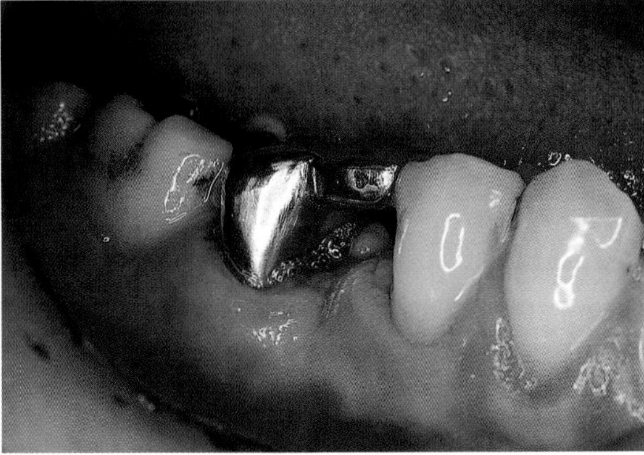

Fig. 3.15 Example of a hygienic pontic.

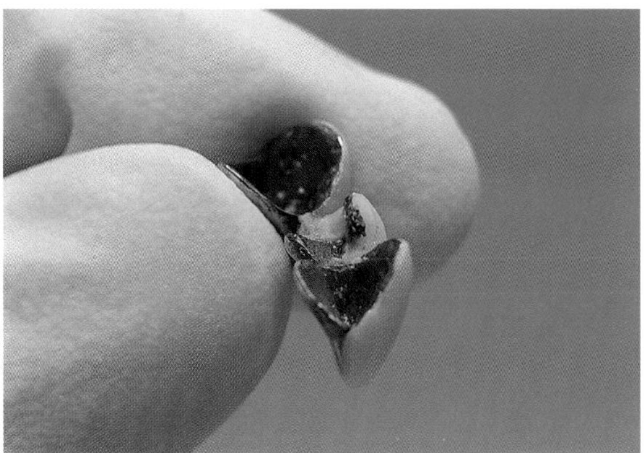

Fig. 3.16 Example of a ridge-lap pontic.

sue contact reduces the amount of 'bubbling' of saliva that can occur between the pontic and gingival tissues during speech.

- *The bullet pontic.* This form is often used in molars or lower incisor situations where the appearance at the gingival margin is not a significant concern. This design has minimal tissue contact and is therefore potentially less retentive of plaque and less likely to lead to gingival irritation (Fig. 3.14).
- *The 'hygienic' or washthrough pontic.* This form (Fig. 3.15) is only very occasionally used and tends to be solely in the lower posterior segments. It is generally associated with all-metal bridgework, solely to restore function. It is an extreme form of open embrasure and is designed to allow the patient to clean the area most effectively.
- *The ridge lap pontic.* This type should be avoided because of its concave tissue contact profile that renders it virtually impossible to clean adequately. According to Fayyad and Al-Rafee (1966), this form of pontic has been associated with designs that have higher failure rates (Fig. 3.16).

Factors relating to long-span bridgework

The flexibility of a beam may be predicted via the following equation:

$$\textbf{Flexibility} = \frac{\textbf{PL}^3}{\textbf{EDW}^3}$$

where P = load applied, L = length of span, E = modulus of elasticity, D = dimension perpendicular to the applied load, and W = dimension parallel to the applied load.

As mentioned earlier, doubling the length of a bridge will effectively lead to an eightfold increase in its flexibility, and this will impart more stress on the luting cement. Occasionally, the flexibility of the metal infrastructure may result in delamination of the porcelain coating. In consequence, shorter units are preferred; they also have the advantage of being easier to remove and/or remake.

As also mentioned previously, there is an increased risk of distortion of long castings during fabrication, and a potential worsening of this following the application of porcelain and its subsequent contraction during firing. One technique that reduces the consequences of this is 'post-ceramic soldering'. This is a technically demanding process that involves an additional clinical stage. Following construction of the bridgework in separate units, these are tried-in in the mouth and a 'pick-up' impression is taken using a non-expansion plaster. The technician uses this impression to place refractory dies and to base the model, orientating the bridge components in the same relationship as that found intraorally. The bridgework units can then be soldered together with minimal distortion, ensuring a passive fit (Wise, 1995).

Factors relating to occlusal schemes for pontics/retainers

Because a stated aim of bridgework is to restore function, the occlusal scheme should fulfil this objective. It is therefore recommended that, as part of the planning process, appropriately articulated study casts are examined. This may involve assessment of handheld casts, or the mounting of the casts on a complex articulator (Fig. 3.7); the clinician has to determine which is required.

Maintenance of ICP

A key feature is that intercuspal contact is maintained. This ensures that the opposing teeth will remain in a stable position. In intercuspal position there should be even contact between both arches, and this can be verified by the use of shimstock foil. The presence of multiple even contacts will reduce the likelihood of the abutment teeth tilting.

Functional movement

With regards to functional movement, as a general rule restorative materials, other than cast metals, tend to be weak to shearing forces and so it is advisable wherever possible to allow guidance to lateral or protrusive movements to be carried predominantly by natural teeth.

Guidance

Where practicable, the patient's existing occlusal scheme – i.e. group function or canine guidance – should be maintained. However, there are exceptions. A root-filled tooth is weaker as a result of coronal and radicular preparation (see above) and is therefore less able to tolerate significant loading without fracture. Where an abutment tooth for a proposed bridge has been root filled, either with or without a post-retained core, it may be appropriate to modify the occlusal scheme.

Canines as retainers/pontics

In the general population canine guidance may be exhibited either unilaterally or bilaterally. If the canine is either root filled or missing it is preferable to avoid using canine guidance in the prosthesis. This reduces the magnitude of potentially damaging forces exerted, but can risk the introduction of working or non-working interference as a consequence of less posterior disclusion during lateral excursions, with consequences that may include posterior cusp fracture.

Factors relating to choice of material for the occlusal surfaces

Significant factors in the choice of occlusal surface restoration material in bridgework again relate to function and aesthetics. All-ceramic occlusal surfaces are usually preferred by patients, owing to the natural appearance of porcelain. However, precise occlusal forms are difficult for the laboratory to fabricate, and such surfaces are also difficult to adjust and finish before cementation without a try-in at the 'biscuit' stage of fabrication. This is less problematic in a posterior bridge, where canine guidance pre-exists and a conformative approach is being adopted. However, where there is evidence of significant parafunction, or if clinical crown height precludes the tooth reduction required for occlusal porcelain coverage, metal surfaces will provide better function.

Where a bridge retainer is intended to provide the guidance it is best that the guiding surfaces be constructed in metal. This offers several advantages:

- Relatively small amounts of tooth reduction for metal coverage
- A smooth, non-abrasive surface can be produced to minimize wear in the opposing tooth
- Cast metals resist high shearing forces well.

These surfaces are often not visible during normal speech and function and so, although the appearance may not be considered ideal, the final aesthetics are usually acceptable.

Table 3.1 Criteria for articulator selection

Handheld models	*Semiadjustable articulator*
Pre-existing canine guidance (occasionally group function)	Group function/class II div 1
Canine not involved in preparation	Canine as pontic
One or two pontics	Multiple pontics
Stable ICP	Reorganized approach required
Preparation will not affect stability of ICP	Preparation will remove ICP stability *or* last tooth(teeth) in arch to be prepared
Sufficient guidance to length of anteriors exists (anterior bridge)	Custom incisal guidance table required
Handheld models	Semiadjustable articulator

Factors relating to choice of articulator

Although these are generally limited in their ability to reproduce mandibular movements, the following 'rules of thumb' can be followed as a guide in the selection of an articulator for bridge fabrication (Table 3.1).

Principles of preparation

When preparing teeth for a conventional bridge, several apparently conflicting requirements (i.e. mechanical versus biological) have to be reconciled (Table 3.2).

Before commencing any preparation, the path of insertion of the bridge should be decided. After the reduction of the occlusal surfaces, the surface of the tooth that dictates the line of insertion should then be prepared. For relatively inexperienced operators it is often helpful to then prepare corresponding surfaces at one time, i.e. the mesial of one abutment followed by the mesial of the other, etc., as this encourages parallelism of the preparations.

From an ideal periodontal viewpoint, supragingival restoration margins are preferred. However, this is often unrealistic where appearance is important and in cases of short clinical crown length. In these circumstances it is often necessary to finish the preparation just within the gingival crevice. In terms of providing conditions for periodontal health, the contour of the retainer (emergence profile) and the shape of the embrasure spaces are more important than the subgingival placement of a well fitting margin.

Table 3.2 Mechanical and biological factors to consider in tooth preparation

Mechanical requirement	Biological imperative
Removal of sufficient tooth structure to allow construction of the prosthesis without occlusal interference or overbuilding of tooth profile (the emergence angle)	Preservation of as much dentine as possible over the vital pulp
Maximum retention and resistance form (gingival margin to occlusal surface height, surface area of preparation and ideal convergence of 6°)	Avoidance of placement of gingival margins at or beyond the junctional epithelium
Long contact areas for maximum strength of the connector	Open embrasures to allow approximal cleansing

Soft tissue management

Gingival tissues should be healthy prior to bridge preparation. Where this is not the case oral hygiene procedures must be instituted, with the appropriate correction of secondary plaque-retaining factors. This may involve the fabrication of a high-quality provisional restoration to maximize healing. The gingivae should also be manipulated carefully during tooth preparation. Uncontrolled trauma is clinically and biologically unacceptable and may result in gingival recession, which will compromise the aesthetics of the final bridge and will often cause haemorrhage that will interfere with impression procedures.

After tooth preparation, and prior to impression making, the soft tissues should be retracted to allow a clear impression of the preparation margins.

A variety of haemorrhage control/gingival retraction procedures are available:

- Physical
- Thermal (electrical)
- Chemical.

Physical retraction usually employs gingival retraction cord. A number of techniques are available, but all aim to widen the gingival crevice and allow the margins to be reproduced. Haemorrhage is controlled by the pressure exerted within the crevice, closing the capillaries. Unfortunately, removal of the cord is often associated with profuse bleeding. This led to the development of the 'twin-cord technique', where one cord is placed deep within the gingival crevice and a larger, more superficial one is then placed. This latter cord only is removed prior to impression procedures and the deeper cord holds the sulcus open and prevents bleeding. Using this technique there is seldom a need for chemical haemostatic agents.

Electrocautery serves a dual role whereby the gingival sulcus is widened by an electrode generating sufficient heat locally to produce a controlled tissue burn. This technique can be used to control haemorrhage by cauterizing the gingival capillaries, as well as to provide space for the impression material to enter the sulcus. Care must be taken not to overheat the tissues, or uncontrolled gingival recession may take place after healing (Louca & Davies, 1992). Accordingly, care should be exercised if there are any underlying dehiscences or the buccal tissues appear particularly 'thin', as is often the case overlying upper canines.

Chemical agents often involve the use of astringents to control haemorrhage. Unless used in conjunction with a retraction cord, they usually offer little help in exposing the gingival margins of preparations.

The most commonly available materials are astringents such as ferric sulphate or aluminium chloride. These act by promoting haemostasis (via their effects on the coagulation cascade), shrinkage of the gingivae and control of crevicular moisture.

Adrenaline – or, more appropriately, noradrenaline – may be used, as this causes constriction of the capillary openings via smooth muscle contraction and therefore controls bleeding, but significant amounts of adrenaline may enter the circulation, and this is often contraindicated in patients with complex medical histories (Donovan et al., 1985)

Newer haemostatic gels have been developed that aim to control haemorrhage within the crevice. These also expand in contact with fluid within the gingival sulcus, providing some retraction of the gingivae. A drawback of these materials is their relative expense and their often unpleasant taste.

Impression technique(s)

With an increased awareness of infection control, which has the potential to affect the impression material and the resultant cast, the use of elastomeric impression materials has predominated over reversible hydrocolloids. Addition-cured polyvinylsiloxane materials are considered the most reliable for fixed prosthodontics because of their dimensional stability. These materials also come in a variety of viscosities and delivery systems that allow the clinician to choose the system that suits them best. The 'one-stage' impression technique (Pameijer, 1983) minimizes the thickness of the light-bodied material (which, because of its low filler content, is most likely to undergo dimensional changes) while providing good surface reproduction.

The most appropriate impression tray material is open to debate but, in vivo, the movement of teeth within the periodontal ligament is a greater confounding factor than any flexibility of polycarbonate trays (Al-Somadi et al., 2001). It is, however, crucial that an appropriate adhesive is used to aid retention of the material within the tray.

Provisional restorations

The functions of the provisional (temporary) bridge are the same as those of the definitive restoration: it should restore function and aesthetics, provide comfort by protecting the pulp (usually in the form of dentinal coverage), and maintain the position of the teeth (abutments and antagonists) following the recording of working impressions.

The construction of the provisional bridge may take place in the laboratory or at the chairside.

Laboratory procedures

This requires the use of preoperative study models that are, ideally, duplicated. One set of models is used for the construction of a diagnostic wax-up and a subsequent silicone putty index. The other is then modified to approximate the required tooth preparation, poly(methyl)methacrylate placed in the silicone index, and the two brought together. The temporary bridge resin material can then be heat-cured to provide an aesthetic and durable provisional.

A significant shortcoming of this technique is that if the models are prepared more radically than the corresponding natural teeth, the provisional restoration will not 'seat' over the preparations and the temporary bridge may require considerable adjustment to allow it to fit. A solution to this is to 'underprepare' the model to leave a thin framework of the provisional bridge that can be relined at the chairside with a suitable material, such as butyl methacrylate, prior to temporary cementation. In extreme circumstances where the use of a provisional restoration may be prolonged, more durable materials may be used. In this situation cast silver may be used for posterior restorations, or silver/acrylic provisional restorations in anterior areas of the mouth.

Clinical procedures

A preoperative diagnostic wax-up may be used to construct a silicone putty index at the chairside, or alternatively a denture tooth may be trimmed and placed into the edentulous space prior to making the index. Following tooth preparation this index can be filled with a suitable material such as a bis-acryl or butyl methacrylate and the index then placed intraorally.

A significant shortcoming of this technique is that certain aspects of the natural tooth will not always be heavily prepared, leading to very thin areas of the provisional material that are prone to fracture. Use of an additional, sectioned preoperative index will ensure that adequate tooth reduction has been performed (Shillingburg et al., 1987.)

An important aspect of the provisional restoration is a precise marginal fit without undue overcontouring at the gingival margin. Any excess in this area may retract the gingivae in the short term and will encourage plaque accumulation, with possible gingival recession in the longer term. This may result in a poor appearance of the final bridge as a result of the margins becoming supragingival.

Try-in

The fabrication of fixed bridge prostheses is complex and parallels that of removable dentures, and so it is surprising that fewer clinicians employ metal, and subsequent ceramic 'biscuit bake' try-ins to refine any occlusal discrepancies and assess the aesthetics prior to finishing the bridgework. This stage also allows the clinician to confirm the absence of any undercuts on the preparation and check the fit for passivity and marginal integrity.

If the bridge is found to be unstable (i.e. it 'rocks') when tried in the patient's mouth, one should check whether this occurs on the model or only in mouth. Common causes of such instability are:

- Temporary cement retained on abutments
- Overbuilt contact points (often due to damage to the model during die-sectioning)
- Damaged dies that no longer correspond with the tooth preparations
- Non-parallel preparations.

It is often worth assessing very critically the quality of preparations and impressions of any bridge, found to rock at try-in, that cannot be resolved by correcting of obvious errors on the fitting surface. If a new impression is required it is almost always of value to refine the preparations beforehand to ensure the greatest chance of success in the subsequent remake.

Temporary cementation

Many clinicians advocate placing the final bridge with a non-setting temporary material, as this allows the aesthetics, fit and occlusion to be assessed over a longer period (Pameijer, 1985). It is important to stress that commonly used zinc-oxide eugenol temporary cements are not suitable for temporary cementation under a well-fitting definitive bridge as, in a thin film thickness under a rigid structure, this will prove almost impossible to remove but will allow leakage in the long term as a result of dissolution. These cements may, however, be used when a modifier is added, as the modifier plasticizes and weakens the cement.

Final cementation should take place when the operator and the patient are both satisfied with the aesthetics, occlusion and function of the bridgework.

Final cementation or luting

Diaz-Arnold et al. (1999) reviewed the commonly available materials for final cementation. There are a number of acceptable luting materials, but the cement with the longest clinical usage is zinc-phosphate cement. This material is known to form a suitably thin film thickness, but its use on freshly cut dentine has been questioned owing to its acidity. The buffering capacity of even thin layers of dentine, however, effectively neutralizes this effect (Wang & Hume, 1988).

All major groups of luting cements achieve relatively high compressive strengths, and these values are often quoted by the manufacturers in advertising media. It should be borne in mind that the failure of luting cements is usually due to shear or tensile forces, and most conventional cements are weak in these respects.

Composite resin luting cements are physically strong in both compression and tension, and they are increasingly finding use in the final cementation of fixed prostheses. Their strength can prove a problem, however, if the bridgework is to be subsequently replaced, owing to their ability to bond via micromechanical retention. This may necessitate the protracted sectioning of separate, but bonded, elements of bridgework from the underlying abutment teeth, compared to the cutting of a groove within, and flexure of, a retainer to fracture the underlying luting cement.

Clinical aspects of cementation

When the bridge is being placed it is important to clean the embrasures and underside of the pontic of cement. Floss placed around a connector before the bridge is cemented will allow these areas to be cleaned immediately after the bridge is cemented. The placement of petroleum jelly underneath the pontic also facilitates this procedure.

After cementation, the patient should be shown how to clean the prosthesis and surrounding tissues using a toothbrush, floss and any other oral hygiene aids that are considered necessary.

Review

Cementation of a bridge should never be considered the ultimate procedure, as the patient must enter a review and maintenance programme. All abutment margins should be reviewed regularly for caries and the bridge itself checked for any failure of the cement lute. This is particularly necessary where the bridge has more than one abutment. By pulling and pushing against the retainer, any failure of the cement lute might be visualized by the creation of 'bubbling' at the margins (Fig. 3.17).

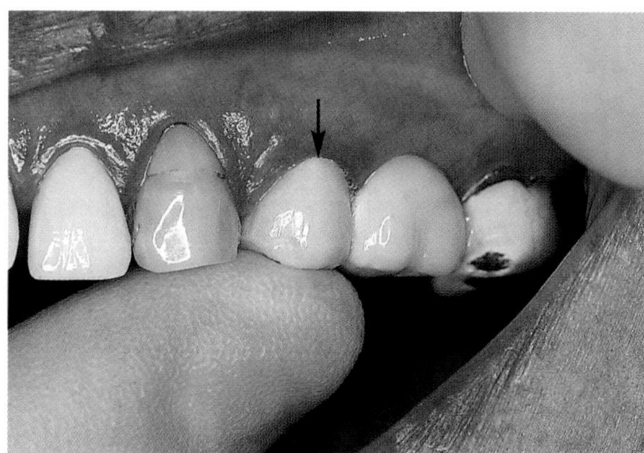

Fig. 3.17 A bubbling effect has been created by testing the stability of the bridge (arrowed).

Another advantage of review appointments is that, even if the bridge continues to function well, the patient's ability to maintain oral hygiene is assessed by the clinician.

RESIN-BONDED BRIDGEWORK

Resin-bonded bridges have become popular as a means of providing a fixed restoration for missing teeth without the amount of tooth preparation required for more conventional designs. It is important to realize, however, that the planning and design stages are just as important and as involved as when full-coverage designs are being used. Appropriate case selection is fundamentally important if this form of prosthesis is to have a reasonable chance of success (Hussey & Wilson, 1999; Morgan et al., 2001).

The failure rate of some resin-bonded bridges has been reported to be as high as 50%, although simple cantilever designs are apparently more successful than fixed–fixed designs (Hussey & Linden, 1996; Botelho, 2000) and anterior bridges are more successful than posterior. Upper bridges have been reported to be more successful than lower bridges (Kellett et al., 1994). The best prognosis, therefore, would appear to be associated with maxillary anterior bridges employing a cantilever design. The use of grooves and rests also appears to provide enhanced retention and resistance form.

As the tooth is minimally prepared, maintaining as much enamel as possible for the most predictable retention employing composite resin cements, these bridges are ideal for young patients with relatively unrestored teeth. The minimal nature of these preparations considerably reduces the morbidity associated with conventional bridgework.

The success of resin-bonded bridges, however, is limited in cases where the abutments are heavily restored, where multiple pontics (more than two) are required, or where excessive force from parafunction or an unfavourable occlusal relationship (e.g. a Class 2 div ii malocclusion) is likely to arise.

Fixed–fixed resin-bonded bridges are considered to have a higher failure rate than cantilever designs, owing to the tendency for the abutment teeth to move in slightly different directions (differential movement) during loading. As the preparation for resin-retained bridgework does not involve complete circumferential reduction (as there is in conventional crown preparation), there is also a tendency for the retainers to be subjected to tensile or shear forces and this stresses the tooth–cement interface. In the case of simple cantilever bridges, the pontic can move slightly with the abutment tooth, no differential movement occurs and the cement lute remains intact.

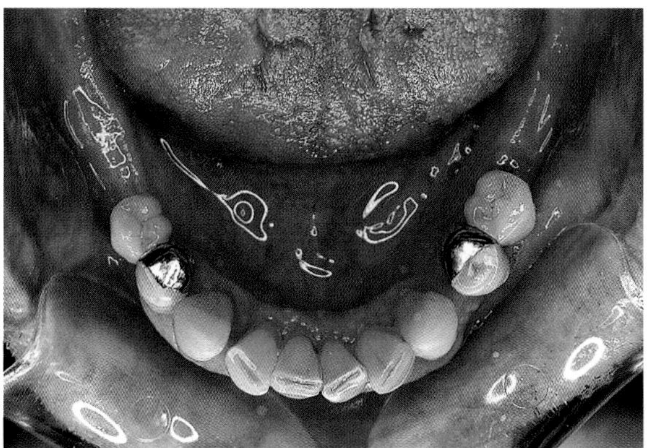

Fig. 3.18 The support of this resin-bonded bridge is derived from sturdy occlusal rests.

A key aspect of tooth preparation for resin-bonded bridgework is that the preparation extends beyond 180° of the prepared tooth surface. This wraparound greatly increases the resistance to displacement. Further retention and resistance can be gained by virtue of grooves and boxes (Byrne et al., 2001). As with all luting cements, the resin lute is relatively weak to shear forces and therefore support from the bridge should be gained from occlusal or cingulum rests (Fig. 3.18).

For resin-bonded bridgework a chemically curing composite resin is used as the luting agent. As with all composite resins good moisture control is required, and the difficulty of achieving this in the mandible without rubber dam may partly explain the poorer success rates of mandibular resin-retained bridgework.

METALWORK

Base metal alloys (based upon Ni-Cr or Co-Cr) are often used for these restorations and have the advantage of being rigid in relatively thin section (0.3 mm is usually adequate). This can usually be accommodated with very limited tooth preparation, and also has the advantage of forming metal oxides that can be utilized in cementation using a chemically active composite resin (i.e. one containing MDP [methacryloyloxydecyldihydrogen phosphate] or 4-META [4-methacryloyloxyethyl-trimellitic acid]).

The fitting surface of the metal is altered to increase its potential for retention to the composite lute. Several methods have been used, but many laboratories now sandblast the fitting surface of the base metals because of the lesser technique sensitivity. This offers predictably good adhesion and the bridges can easily be modified and re-sandblasted, if necessary, prior to cementation. Electrolytically etched metals require re-etching if they are tried-in before cementation, and this often involves an additional laboratory stage.

Clinical experience suggests that the most common form of failure of a fixed–fixed resin-bonded bridge is the failure of the bond to one of the abutments. In these circumstances the bridge has often been functioning as a cantilever, and the lifespan of the restoration can often be enhanced by sectioning of the debonded retainer from the bridge. This is usually a simple procedure, but it can be difficult to produce a cleansable shape at the sectioned surface to prevent caries from arising in the contact area.

REFERENCES

Academy of Prosthodontics. The glossary of prosthodontic terms, 7th edn. J Prosthet Dent 1999; 81: 39–110

Al-Somadi L, Youngson CC, Bates C. Dimensional stability of elastomeric impression in polycarbonate and stainless steel trays *in vitro* and *in vivo.* J Dent Res 2001; 80: 1162

Botelho M. Design principles for cantilevered resin-bonded fixed partial dentures. Quint Int 2000; 31: 613–619

Byrne D, Hussey D, Claffey N. Effect of groove placement on the retention/resistance of resin-bonded retainers for maxillary and mandibular second molars. J Prosthet Dent 2001; 85: 472–478

Diaz-Arnold AM, Vargas MA, Haselton DR. Current status of luting agents for fixed prosthodontics. J Prosthet Dent 1999; 81: 135–141

Donovan TE, Gandara BK, Memetz H. Review and survey of medicaments used with gingival retraction cords. J Prosthet Dent 1985; 53: 525–531

European Society of Endodontology. Consensus report of European Society of Endodontology on quality guidelines for endodontic treatment. Int Endodont J 1994; 27: 115–124

Fayyad MA, Al-Rafee MA. Failure of dental bridges. II. Prevalence of failure and its relation to place of construction. J Oral Rehab 1996; 23: 438–440

Fayyad MA, Al-Rafee MA. Failure of dental bridges. IV. Effect of supporting periodontal ligament. J Oral Rehab 1997; 24: 401–403

Guzy GE, Nicholls JI. An in vitro comparison of intact endodontically treated teeth with and without endo–post reinforcement. J Prosthet Dent 1979; 42: 39–44

Hämmerle CH, Ungerer MC, Fantoni PC et al. Long-term analysis of biologic and technical aspects of fixed partial dentures with cantilevers. Int J Prosthodont 2000; 13: 409–415

Hussey DL, Linden GJ. The clinical performance of cantilevered resin-bonded bridgework. J Dent 1996; 24: 251–256

Hussey DL, Wilson NHF. The provision of resin-bonded bridgework within the General Dental Services 1987–1997. Prim Dent Care 1999; 6: 21–24

Kellett M, Verzijden CW, Smith GA, Creugers NH. A multicentered clinical study on posterior resin-bonded bridges: the 'Manchester trial'. J Dent 1994; 22: 208–212

Louca C, Davies B. Electrosurgery in restorative dentistry: 2. Clinical applications. Dental Update 1992; 19: 364–368

Morgan C, Djemal S, Gilmour G. Predictable resin-bonded bridges in general dental practice. Dental Update 2001; 28: 501–508

Nayyar A, Walton RE, Leonard LA. An amalgam coronal–radicular dowel and core technique for endodontically treated posterior teeth. J Prosthet Dent 1980; 43: 303–307

Nyman S, Lindhe J. A longitudinal study of combined periodontal and prosthetic treatment of patients with advanced periodontal disease. J Periodontol 1979; 50: 163–169

Pameijer CH. A one-step putty-wash impression technique utilizing vinyl polysiloxanes. Quint Int 1983; 14: 861–863

Pameijer J. Periodontal and occlusal factors in crown and bridge procedures. Amsterdam: Dental Centre for Postgraduate Courses 1985

Potts RG, Shillingburg HT, Duncanson MG. Retention and resistance of preparations for cast restorations. J Prosthet Dent 1980; 43: 303–307

Ramfjord SP. Periodontal aspects of restorative dentistry. J Oral Rehab 1974; 1: 107–126

Randow K, Glantz P-O, Zoger B. Technical failures and some related clinical complications in extensive fixed prosthodontics. Acta Odontol Scand 1986; 44: 533–546

Roberts DH. The relationship between age and the failure rate of bridge prostheses. Br Dent J 1970; 128: 175–177

Saunders WP, Saunders E. Prevalence of periradicular periodontitis associated with crowned teeth in an adult Scottish population. Br Dent J 1998; 185: 137–140

Shillingburg HT, Jacobi R, Brackett SE. Fundamentals of tooth preparations for cast metal and porcelain preparations. Chicago: Quintessance, 1987

Sorrensen JA, Engleman MJ. Effect of ferrule design on fracture resistance of endodontically treated teeth. J Prosthet Dent 1990; 66: 343–347

Wang JD, Hume WR. Diffusion of hydrogen ion and hydroxyl ion from various sources through dentine. Int Endodont J 1988; 6: 21–24

Wise MD. Failure in the restored dentition: management and treatment. Chicago: Quintessence, 1987

4 Considerations for removable prostheses

INTRODUCTION

Once the patient has agreed to the provision of a removable prosthesis, there are a number of factors to consider. In the main, these will be specific for each patient. However, there are some that are general and which relate to clinical common sense. For example, not all prostheses should be considered as 'definitive'. Some are clearly intended to help diagnosis, some to be of short duration, and some for a specific therapeutic purpose. Examples of some of these are given in Table 4.1.

It is perhaps unrealistic to consider any prosthesis as being 'permanent', and in the interests of clarity clinicians ought to be aware of the fact that, on occasions, it is useful to consider prostheses as being:

- Preliminary to definitive treatment, or
- Definitive treatment.

The execution of the design of a removable prosthesis should be thorough, irrespective of its intended duration, and the notion that any prosthesis 'is only a temporary denture' is to be deprecated.

To avoid repetition, this chapter will deal with the planning processes for removable prostheses in broad terms, and the considerations for all of the categories of prostheses listed in Table 4.1 will be covered under one umbrella.

Table 4.1 Types of prosthesis according to their intended purpose

Intended nature of prosthesis	Example
Diagnostic	Occlusal splints (? 'bite-freeing')
Short duration	Immediate-insertion prostheses Training dentures Manchester veneers (McCord et al., 1992)
Therapeutic	Training plates for patients who retch
Definitive	Any prosthesis intended to be in place for more than 6 months without any required reline or addition

STAGES IN PLANNING REMOVABLE PROSTHESES

Outlining the saddles

When the factors listed in Chapter 2 have been considered and the agreed option is a removable prosthesis, the clinician has to decide which of the missing teeth are to be replaced and which saddles are to be restored. For example, in Figure 4.1a, there is only one saddle and one tooth to be replaced (albeit for a short time) with a removable prosthesis; this part of the decision-making process is relatively straightforward. In Figure 4.1b, there are several teeth to be replaced and several saddles. Not all of the teeth and not all of the saddles *need* to be replaced, as this might result in unnecessary tooth involvement with the denture and, in addition, may compromise appearance and retention (see below). In Figure 4.1c, however, no teeth may be being replaced but, as an occlusal splint is required, the prosthesis will cover an entire dental arch. The decision to restore a saddle or not will inevitably simplify or complicate the design, as has been referred to above.

Most textbooks on removable partial prosthodontics suggest that this stage of the denture design process should be performed as the commencement of a logical sequence. This has much merit as a teaching or training method, but in reality the decision on whether to restore an edentulous area ought to have been made concurrent with the decision of how to restore the missing tooth/teeth. We consider that all graduate clinicians ought to be aware of the need to plan holistically, and that it is good practice to formulate a tentative denture design concurrent with the formulation of the treatment plan. In this way, the three clinical options illustrated in Figure 4.1 may be made at the chairside; the clinician may alter the design after reflective thought, and having the benefit of articulated casts and following thorough cast analysis. The latter makes ultimate sense, as no prosthesis should be planned without considering the patient's intermaxillary relationships: sometimes, for example, there is no space for a prosthesis, and a predefinitive stage may be required (Fig. 4.2).

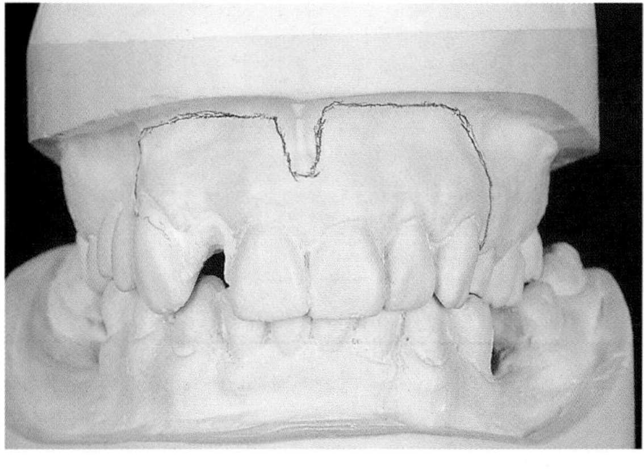

a

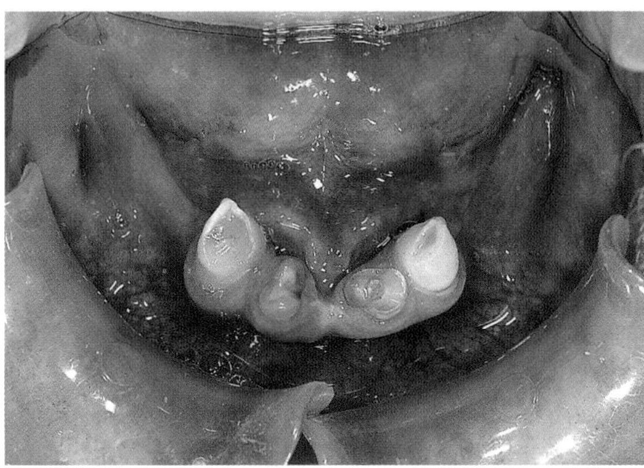

b

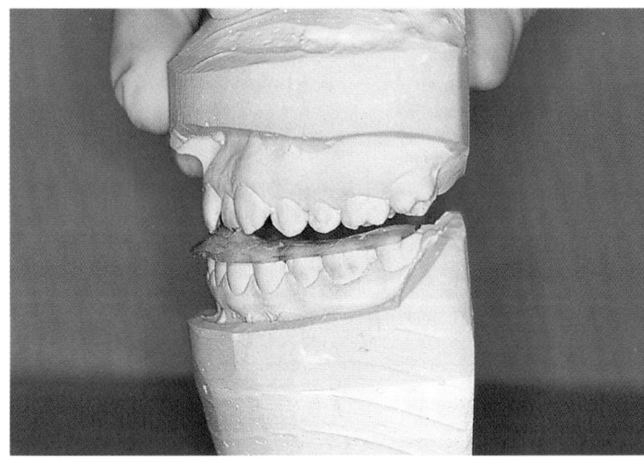

c

Fig. 4.1 (a) This maxillary cast has one edentulous area and one tooth is missing from that area. (b) There are several edentulous areas and some have more than one tooth missing. (c) No teeth are missing here, but a prosthesis has been prescribed to serve as a splint.

Deciding on the nature of the support

Over the years, a variety of clinicians have offered suggestions for classifications of dentures based on support. For any classification to be useful, it should be:

- Consistent

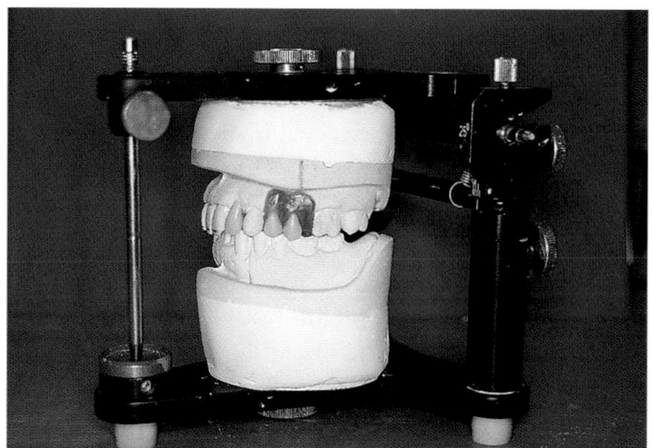

Fig. 4.2 The articulated casts should be examined to check for available space.

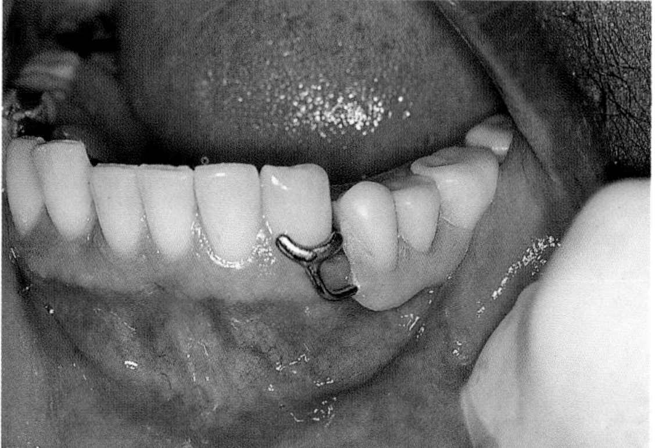

Fig. 4.3 This mandibular denture is tissue-borne and has 'sunk' into the tissues.

- Unambiguous
- Generally accepted.

According to Osborne and Lammie (1974), however, a classification of partial dentures should do more than the above and ought to suggest the main problem involved in the particular case. For this reason no one classification is ideal, and perhaps the most useful is that outlined, in one form or another, by Beckett (1953), Craddock (1956) and Osborne and Lammie (1974):

- Class I: Denture supported by mucosa and underlying bone
- Class II: Denture supported by teeth
- Class III: Denture supported by a combination of mucosa and tooth-borne means.

We consider that this classification should now be extended to include a further type, namely:

- Class IV: Denture supported by implants (see Chapter 5).

It must be realized that this classification is not ranked in order of precedence but could perhaps be considered in order of complexity of planning. For this reason, the support options will be discussed in the above order.

Class 1 Dentures (deriving their support from mucosa and underlying bone)

Wills and Manderson (1977) and Picton and Wills (1978) clarified some misconceptions on the displacement and deformation properties of oral mucosa with their research on primates. They determined that the effects of loading mucosa over a long period were to compress it by up to 45% of its original thickness and, further, that its recovery was viscoelastic in nature. These findings were confirmed by the research of Kydd and Daly (1982). The time required for recovery from the displacing forces has also been found to increase with age. What this clearly means, however, is that prostheses which derive their support from mucosa and the underlying bone will inevitably do two things:

- Displace mucosa
- Result in further loss of alveolar bone (this is perhaps of greater importance).

From the above, it is clear that in mandibular dentures especially, mucosa-borne partial prostheses ought to be considered as a last resort, or possibly as a transitional phase to complete dentures (Fig. 4.3). More latitude exists in the maxilla, however, where the hard palate affords additional support, but this is often abused (Fig. 4.4).

Class II Dentures (deriving their support from teeth)

Tooth-supported prostheses gain their support from the teeth via the supreme qualitative and quantitative support agent, namely the periodontal membrane. Pressure down the long axis of the tooth imparts tension in the periodontal

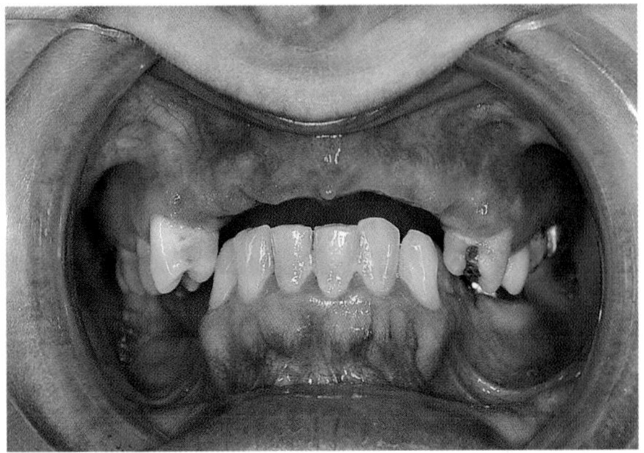

Fig. 4.4 Poor planning of the upper denture has resulted in gum-stripping. An added complication was that the opposing teeth erupted, causing major problems of space.

membrane, which in turn helps to maintain alveolar bone. Clearly this is the most desirable form of support and should be used whenever practicable. It has traditionally been taught that dentures may gain tooth support from incisal rests, occlusal rests or cingulum rests. This reflects on less holistic prosthodontics than may be currently practised, and Table 4.2 suggests a more detailed outline of tooth-derived support.

The statements in the foregoing paragraph indicate that, theoretically, support derived from teeth is more desirable than any other single form of support, and this is a scientifically established fact. However, on occasion the clinician has a need to be empirical and to prescribe what is most appropriate for the patient. For example, a patient who has been treated for chronic periodontal disease may have lost considerable bony support, and a cast metal framework utilizing occlusal rests and cast cobalt chromium clasp assemblies may impart inappropriate forces on a tooth (see pp 42–44).

It should be redundant to state that there is no place nowadays for wrought occlusal rests – they cannot offer an acceptably accurate fit and therefore cannot transfer occlusal loads in a satisfactory manner.

Class III Dentures (deriving their support from a combination of mucosa and tooth-borne means)

It is perhaps no coincidence that clinicians and patients alike have embraced the shortened dental arch philosophy. The option to do nothing or to

Table 4.2 Possible means of tooth support

Details of tooth support	Description
Occlusal rest	Typically a saucer-shaped depression in a natural tooth prepared to house a metal casting, although if a parallelometer is used a metal/metalloceramic crown may be waxed-up to receive a wedged-box inlay preparation (Figs 4.5a and b)
Incisal rest	Less common nowadays, as most western European and North American patients do not find the appearance acceptable (Fig. 4.6)
Cingulum rest	A common supporting element which has the double advantage of providing good reciprocation to a direct retainer on the same tooth. Typically, this is created through the use of a tapered fissure bur and presents a positive ledge in the cingulum (Fig. 4.7). Cingulum rests may also be created or acquired via adhesive techniques, when composite resin or a metal alloy may be added to the surface of a tooth
Milled crown	Offers the potential for good support down the long axis of the supporting tooth and, if planned well, prevents coverage of the gingivae by the major connector (Fig. 4.8)
Overdenture	May be a decoronated tooth, which has usually undergone endodontic treatment. May or may not have a precision attachment on or in the root face

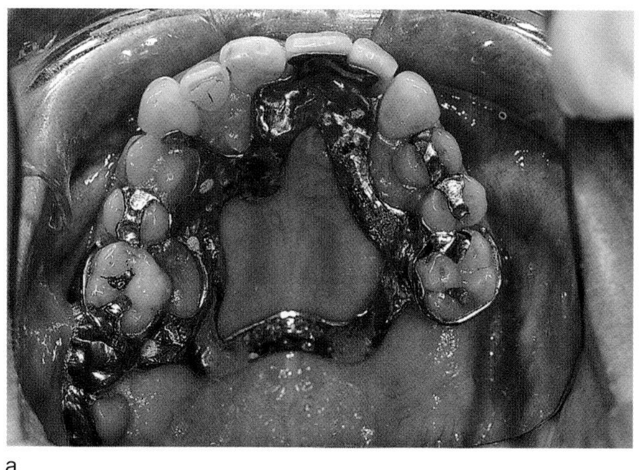

a

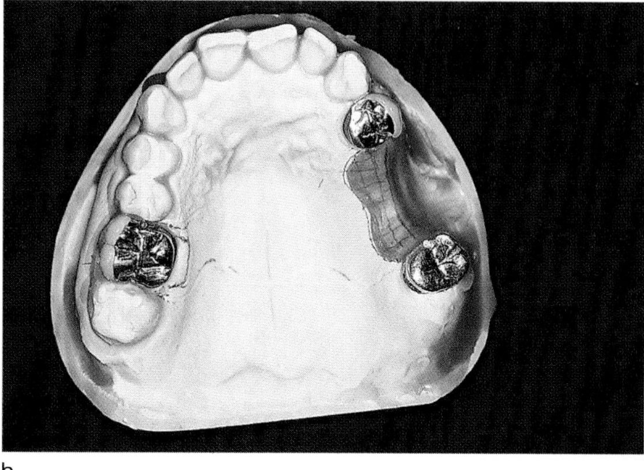

b

Fig. 4.5 (a) Form of occlusal rests on abutment teeth to provide occlusal contact and engender stability to the denture. (b) Milled occlusal rests on crowned abutment teeth.

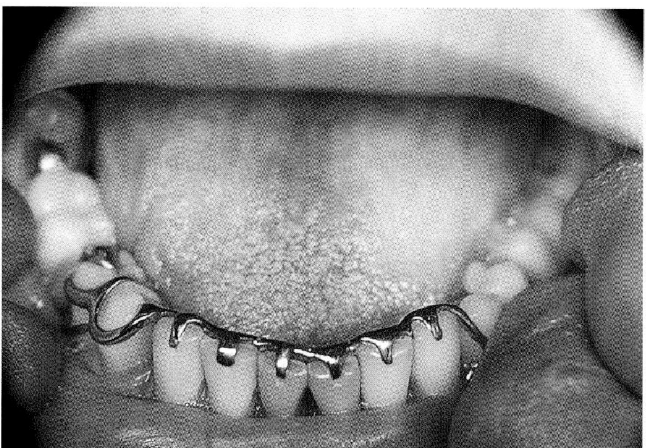

Fig. 4.6 Incisor rests have been included in this denture but the appearance has been compromised.

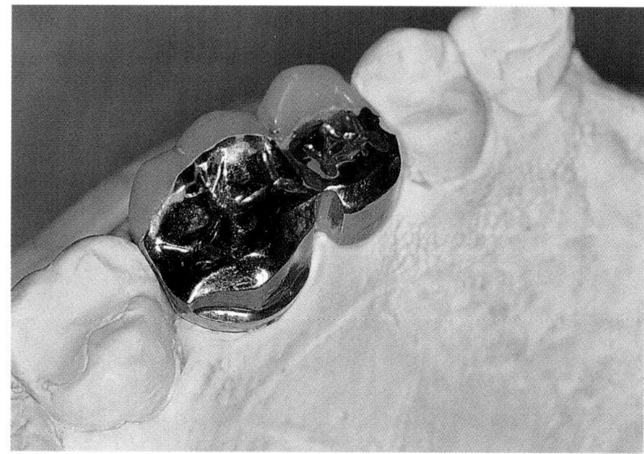

Fig. 4.8 Milled crown, shoulder clear.

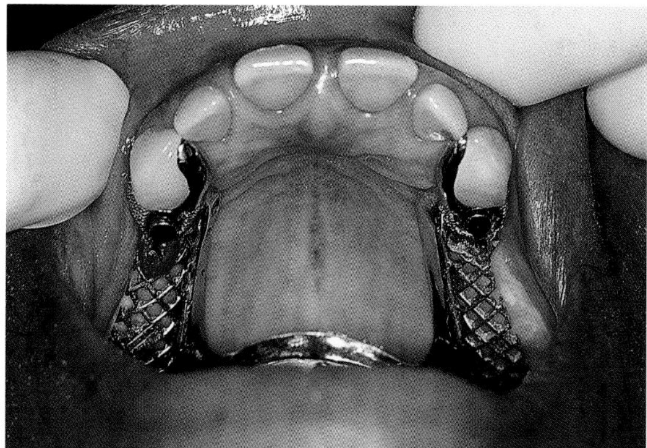

Fig. 4.7 Cingulum rests have been milled to fit into a shoulder on the crowns of the canines.

use a fixed prosthesis to replace one dental unit (e.g. by cantilevering one unit from the terminal abutment) is seen as being less problematic than providing a removable prosthesis to replace several missing teeth. From the clinician's viewpoint this is because of the very real and problematic differences between the two supporting elements, and from the patient's perspective because of intensive tissue coverage.

Extrapolating the results of Wills and Manderson (1977) and Wills et al. (1980), the clear fact emerges that, long after abutment teeth have returned to their resting positions (after mastication, for example), the mucosa will remain displaced; this displacement is of the order of 20 times that of the teeth even on the basis of a maximally covered saddle. It will be self-evident to state that mucosa under minimally covered saddles will be displaced even more than under maximally covered saddles.

This support differential is thus problematic, and the inherent tendency for a prosthesis to demonstrate rocking (instability) has resulted in philosophies of clasping which were based on homeostatic principles of stress-breaking, whereas others were based on more biological principles (Kratochvil, 1963; Krol, 1973). The 1983 Symposium on Restoration of the Partially Dentate Mouth (Bates et al., 1984) effectively refuted the stress-breaker concept, and the philosophy of clasping in this type of prosthesis is now more biologically friendly (see below). Another complicating factor to bear in mind, arising from the disparity in the supporting agents, is the need to consider antirotation devices, and this will also be considered later.

Class IV Dentures (deriving their support from implants)

Implant-supported prostheses will be considered in Chapter 5.

Deciding on the form of the major connector

As presented in many textbooks, the next stage of the design process is to consider how the prosthesis will be retained. It became clear in the planning stages of this book that the authors tend to consider the major connector next, and thus we offer this as the next stage of the design of the removable prosthesis. Just as in a fixed prosthesis, where the bounded saddle is restored with a tooth/teeth forming the pontic, so in a removable prosthesis we use a component called not a pontic but a major connector. This must be rigid and capable of transferring occlusal and masticatory loads to the supporting elements of the denture without adversely affecting these denture-bearing tissues. The types of major connector in common use are listed in Table 4.3.

These are merely descriptions of the form of the component. The decision on the nature of the material (from which the connector is produced) must be based on the clinical findings and the future needs of the patient. If the prosthesis is intended to be an immediate denture, or if it is to be a splint to treat temporomandibular dysfunction symptoms, then the material of choice will invariably be poly(methyl)methacrylate (PMMA). If smaller areas of coverage are intended and the major connector is required to be intrinsically strong, then a metal alloy is indicated. The most common alloy in clinical usage is cobalt-chromium, although type IV gold alloys may be used. More recently, titanium alloys have been recommended, but the technical requirements of the latter are more rigorous than the former two, and so more

Table 4.3 Common major connectors

Maxillary	Mandibular
Palatal plate (Fig. 4.9)	Lingual plate (Fig. 4.15)
Palatal strap (Fig. 4.10)	Lingual bar (Fig. 4.16)
Anterior or posterior palatal bar (Fig. 4.11)	Sublingual bar (Fig. 4.17)
Skeletal design (Fig. 4.12)	Kennedy bar, i.e. a lingual bar plus a continuous clasp (Fig. 4.18)
Horseshoe design (Fig. 4.13)	Labial bar
Labial bar (Fig. 4.14)	

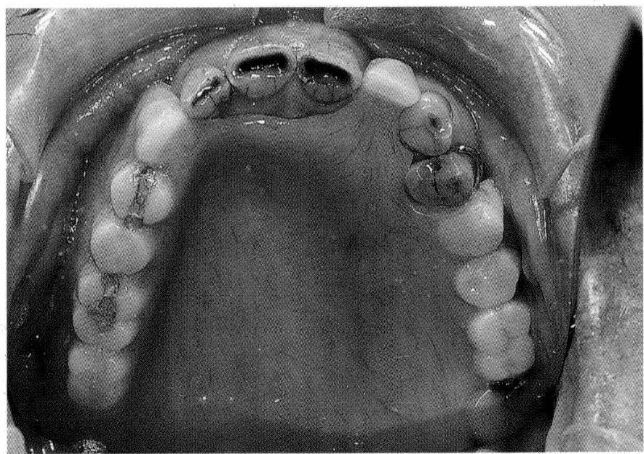

Fig. 4.9 Palatal plate.

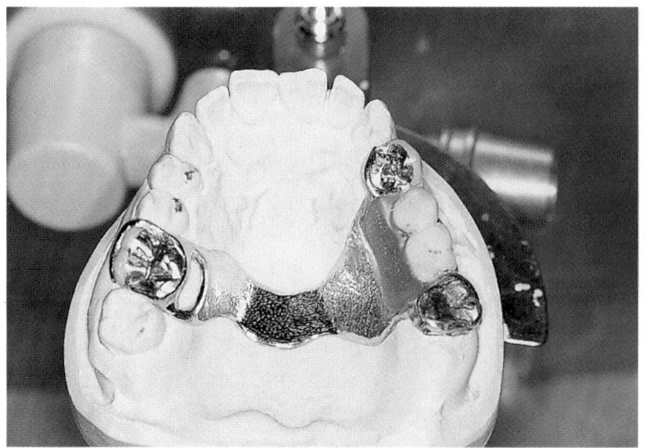

Fig. 4.10 Palatal strap.

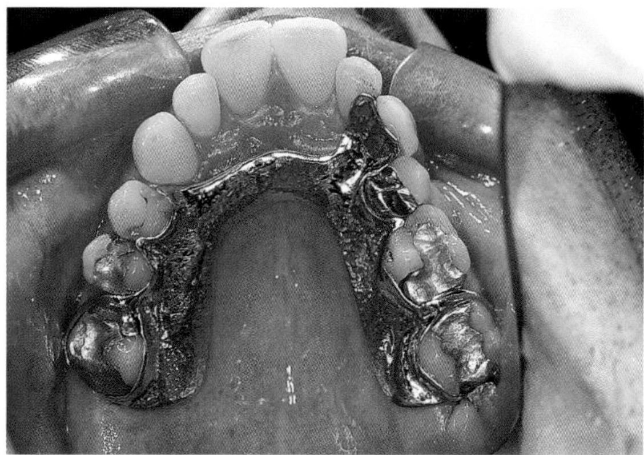

Fig. 4.13 Horseshoe design.

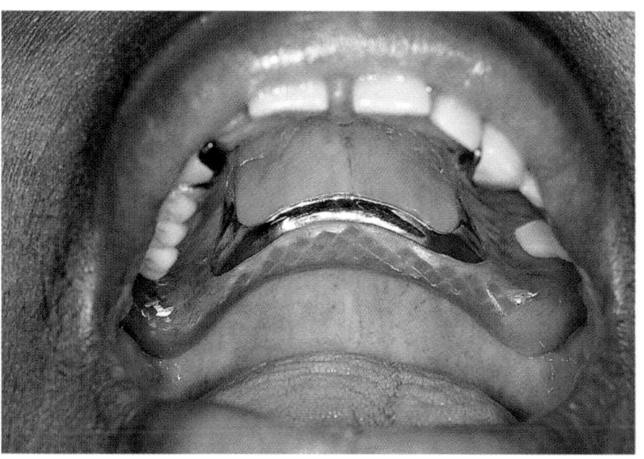

Fig. 4.11 Posterior palatal bar.

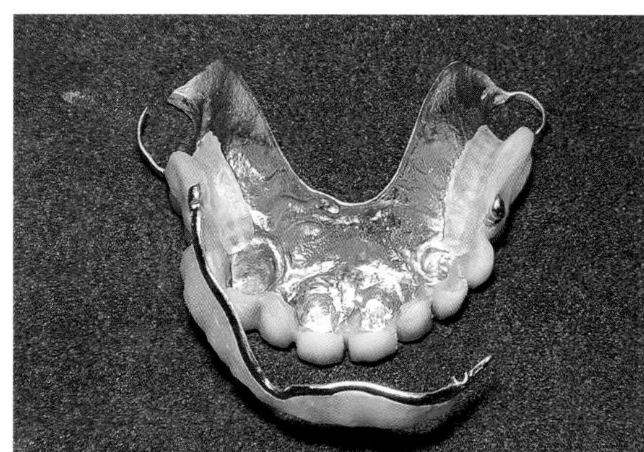

Fig. 4.14 Labial bar.

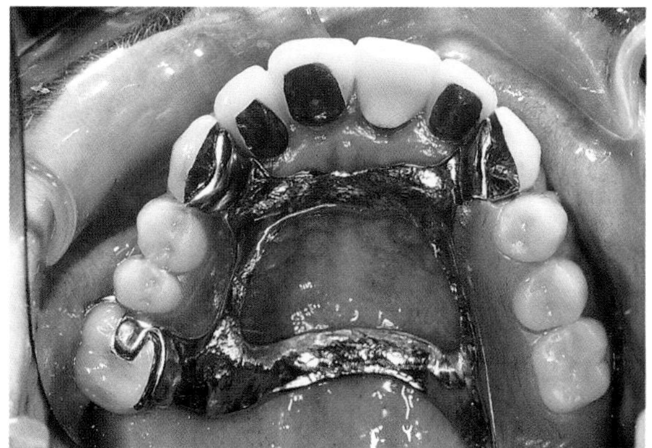

Fig. 4.12 Skeletal design.

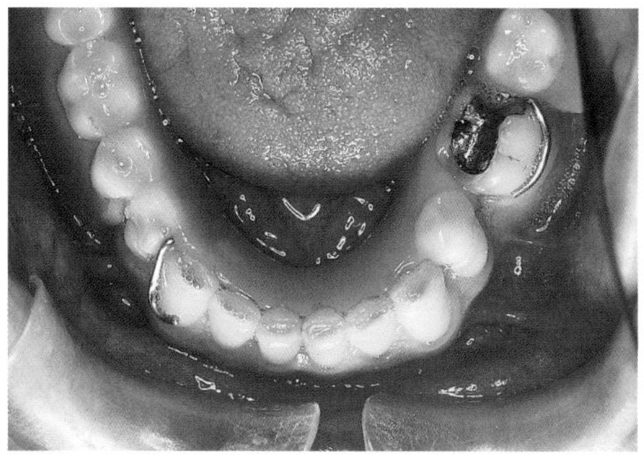

Fig. 4.15 Lingual plate.

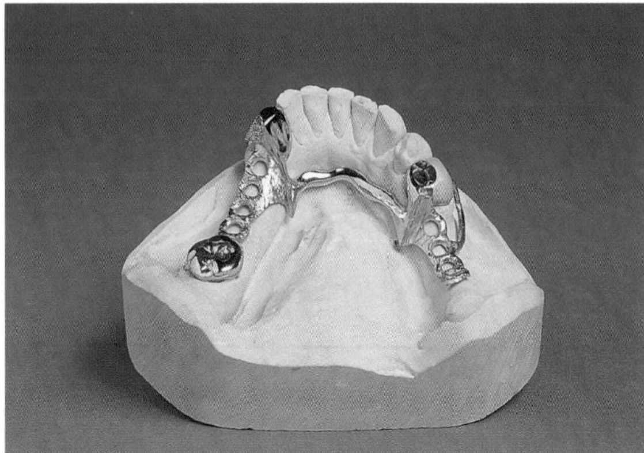

Fig. 4.16 Lingual bar.

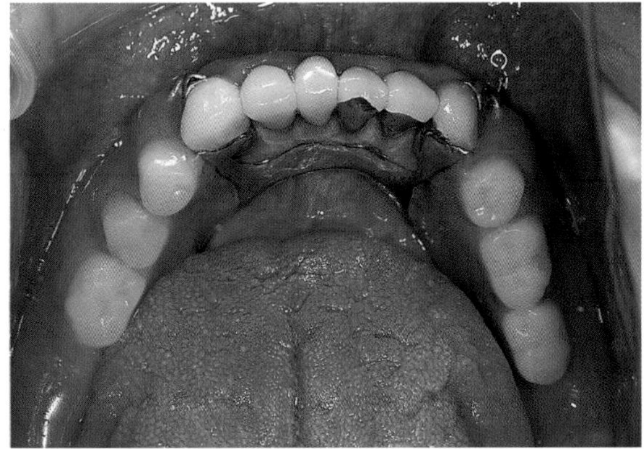

Fig. 4.17 Sublingual bar.

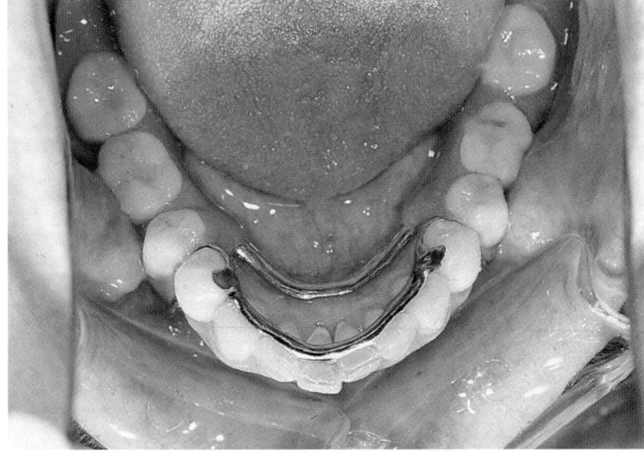

Fig. 4.18 Kennedy bar.

clinical testing is required before they enjoy the popularity of the cobalt-chromium alloys.

Deciding on how the prosthesis will be retained

Irrespective of whether it is to be fixed or removable, the clinician must plan to ensure that the prosthesis resists movement away from the tissues that support it. Fixed prostheses gain support from the height and 'parallelism' of the abutment tooth preparations plus the cement/luting material. In the case of removable prostheses, retention is achieved in a variety of ways, and these are listed in Table 4.4. Not included here is neuromuscular control, principally because this is not quantifiable; nor can it be guaranteed that all patients develop it well.

Although some patients are able to control their dentures without the aid of any retainer or adhesive, we do not consider that any clinician can provide a prosthesis without direct retainers and be confident that it will be adequately retained. Equally, it is generally considered that it

Table 4.4 Direct retainers

Type of direct retainer	Clinical examples
Clasps	Gingivally approaching Occlusally approaching
Precision attachments	Intracoronal attachment Extracoronal attachment Studs Bars Others
Planned use of undercuts not on buccal or lingual of teeth	Guide planes Use of bony undercuts, e.g. labial undercuts in anterior bounded saddles
Use of resilient materials	Resilient materials, e.g. silicone rubber to engage undercuts
Denture adhesives	Usually resorted to by patients, but may be suggested by clinician in certain situations

is impossible to attain a peripheral seal (to assist retention) where partial dentures are concerned. However, it is suggested that, in certain situations, the provision of a peripheral seal is possible.

Clasps

The type or form of clasp is generally selected after surveying the cast. Surveying is generally performed at right-angles to the occlusal plane in the first instance, as this is the likely path of displacement. Surveyors are basically simple instruments which enable a cast to be analysed with respect to tooth contour. Not all surveyors are bulky, and the authors recommend that practitioners use a simple one (Fig. 4.19).

Surveying will identify three principal factors:

- The presence of undercuts
- The contour of the undercuts relative to the gingival margin
- The depth of the undercuts.

Clearly, the absence of undercuts will suggest that no direct retention from clasps is available, and some method whereby retention may be achieved needs to be incorporated. This could be done relatively easily by the addition of composite resin

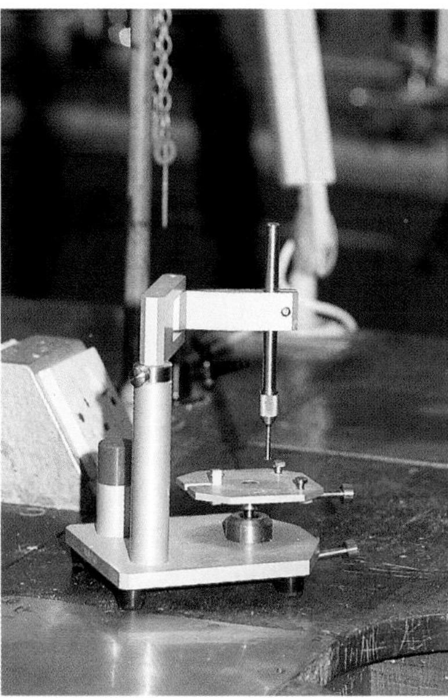

Fig. 4.19 A simple surveyor for surgeries.

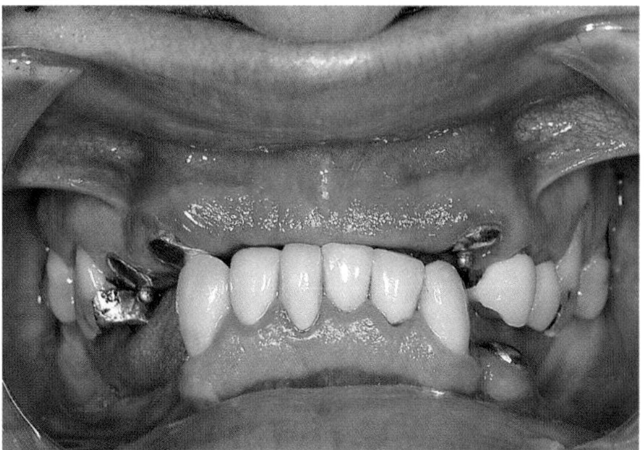

Fig. 4.20 Some composite has been added to the buccal aspect of the lower right canine to provide an undercut.

(Fig. 4.20) or by a crown or, if a crown already exists, by creating a dimple in the crown (Figs 4.21), taking care not to perforate it. The contour of the undercuts relative to the gingivae will determine if the clasp is to be gingivally approaching or occlusally approaching. As the health of the periodontium must not be compromised, it is clear that clasp arms and clasp tips should be clear of the gingival margins of abutment teeth.

The depth of the undercut is determined via undercut gauges, three of which are in current use, namely 0.25 mm, 0.5 mm and 0.75 mm. As all direct retainers, especially clasps, work by making the retaining element deform, the deformation must be controlled, and it is this component that determines, fundamentally, the material used for the direct retainer.

For example, in large undercuts more flexible clasps are required, and these will inevitably be wrought in nature; for 0.25 mm undercuts less flexibility is required and cast cobalt-chromium may be used. However, the clinician should be mindful of the application of biomaterials science when he/she considers the material, and this is particularly relevant here. Bates (1965) and Prabowa (1995) have referred to the need for a minimal length of cast cobalt-chromium for flexibility. This is 14 mm; as no premolar tooth is 14 mm in length mesiodistal, there is no scientific basis for making cast cobalt-chromium clasp arms *which are occlusally approaching* on premolar teeth. If it is not possible to have gingivally approaching

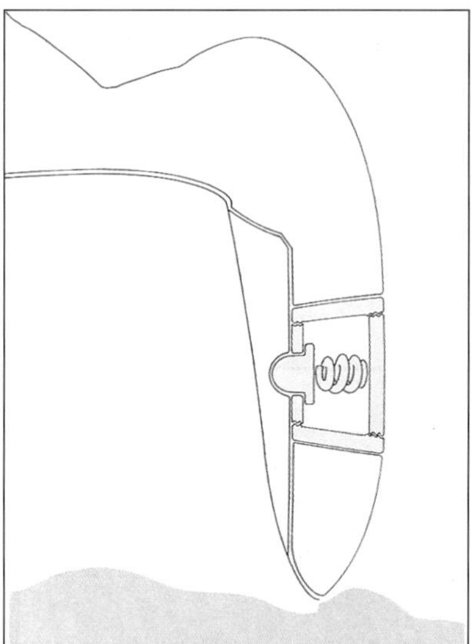

Fig. 4.21 A thimble crown has an indent on the buccal aspect, into which a precision attachment is placed. Alternatively, a clasp arm could be placed into the created undercut.

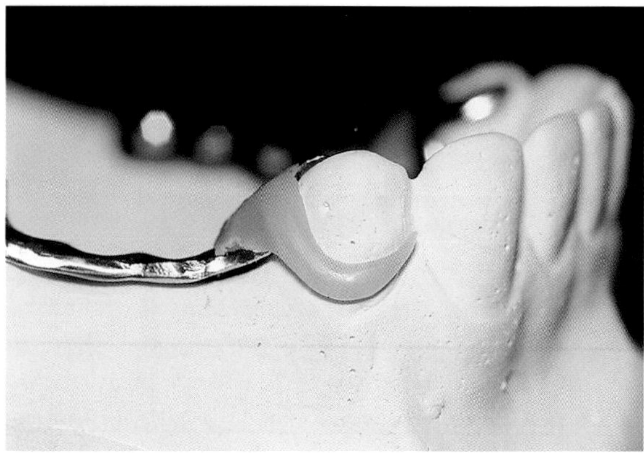

Fig. 4.22 Dental D clasp. Note its proximity to the gingival margin.

clasps then some other form of direct retention is indicated. This is because short clasps tend to deform permanently or to fracture because the elastic deformation of cobalt-chromium in these circumstances is inadequate.

Reference was made earlier to the analysis of articulated casts, and the clinician ought to be aware of the three-dimensional nature of clasp assemblies. This is particularly true when occlusal rests are part of the assembly. Careful analysis of the articulated cast will enable the clinician to see whether there is space for the occlusal rest and/or clasp arms; if no space exists, tooth preparation is required, for which informed consent must be obtained (see Fig. 1.9c).

The importance of appearance should also be considered, and this is why a tooth-coloured polymeric material was introduced (Dental D). It is not clear whether this material demonstrates the desired qualities to act as a direct retainer, and the advantages of its colour should never be to the detriment of the patient's tissues (Fig. 4.22).

Precision attachments

According to *The Glossary of Prosthodontic Terms* (Academy of Prosthodontics, 1999), a precision attachment is: 'a device which comprises of two or more components which is machined or fabricated for the purposes of providing retention to a prosthesis'. Typically, there are five types of precision attachment and they are listed in Table 4.5.

For further details, readers are referred to standard textbooks (e.g. Preiskel, 1979), although further examples of precision attachments will be discussed in the chapter on implant-retained and supported prostheses.

Planned use of undercuts not on buccal or lingual aspects of teeth

Reference has been made to the need to analyse articulated casts and to survey for undercuts at right-angles to the occlusal plane. Unfortunately, certain clinical conditions conspire to complicate planning, and this is particularly true where anterior bounded saddles exist, and also where posterior free-end saddles exist. These situations may result in diminished retention, and they may also reduce the potential for an aesthetic result (Figs 4.31, 4.32). In both cases a second survey is required (giving a dual survey) to eliminate the undercut areas and provide paths of insertion (and thus of withdrawal) which are not the same as the natural path of displacement (Fig. 4.33). In essence, the second survey determines a plane of insertion, and this is termed a **guide plane.** Guide planes may need to be created by inten-

Table 4.5 A simple classification of precision attachments, with examples of each type

Type of precision attachment	Example	General comment
Intracoronal	Pin-slot (Fig. 4.23) Chayes	Inherently requires loss of tooth tissue and needs a minimum of 5 mm height from base of floor of cavity to the marginal ridge
Extracoronal	Ceka (Fig. 4.24) Dalla-bona	May be resilient or non-resilient. Also requires width and height (5 mm)
Stud	Dalbo Rotherman (Fig. 4.25)	Need to be aware of the potential for bulk and to plan common paths of withdrawal
Bar	Dolder-type (Fig. 4.26) Hader-type (Fig. 4.27)	The type of bar used may impart the potential to rotate about the bar axis; space requirements are also important, and if an RPD is being used the wax trial denture should be assessed prior to fabricating the bar
Other	Hinges (Fig. 4.28) Spring-loaded ball (Fig. 4.29) Split-pin and tube (Fig. 4.30)	May be problematic to repair Useful but not for free-end saddles Useful in some sectional denture cases

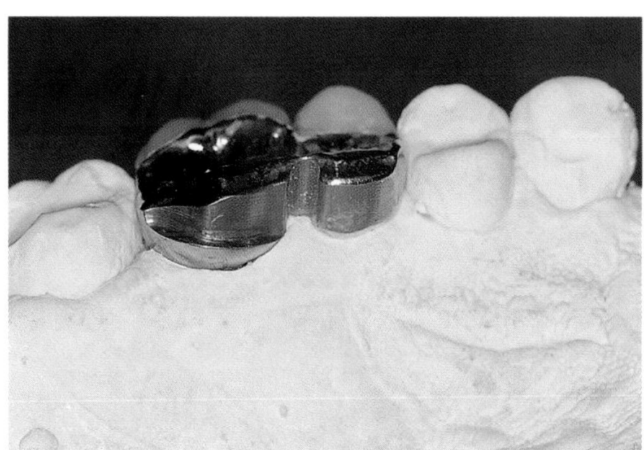

Fig. 4.23 Pin-slot in interproximal grooves.

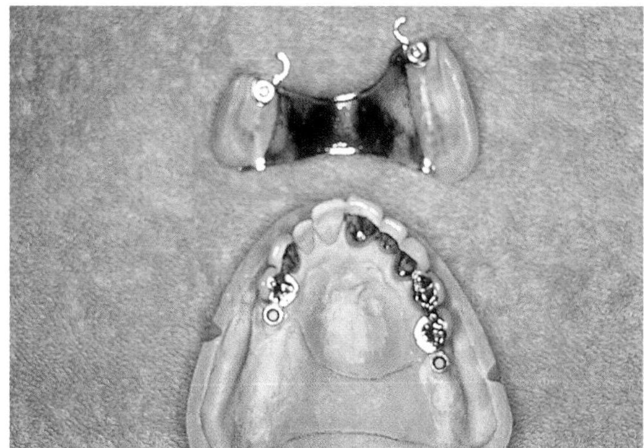

Fig. 4.24 Ceka extracoronal attachment.

tional modification of tooth contour or by planned contour of fixed restorations (Fig. 4.34). This is the basis of the RPI system advocated by Kratochvil (1963), and modified by Krol in 1973, as a solution to the problems of free-end saddles.

R stands for the occlusal rest, which is placed on the mesial of the terminal abutment tooth. **P** stands for the guide plane, which enhances retention and ought to reduce rotating movements on the tooth. **I** stands for the I-bar, which is the principal direct retainer.

Reciprocation for this I-bar, which should be on the distobuccal aspect of the tooth, is achieved via the mesially placed occlusal rest. Again, further details are available in standard textbooks of prosthodontics.

A more sophisticated philosophy concerns a rotational path of insertion. This was reviewed by Krol and Finzen (1988) (Fig. 4.35).

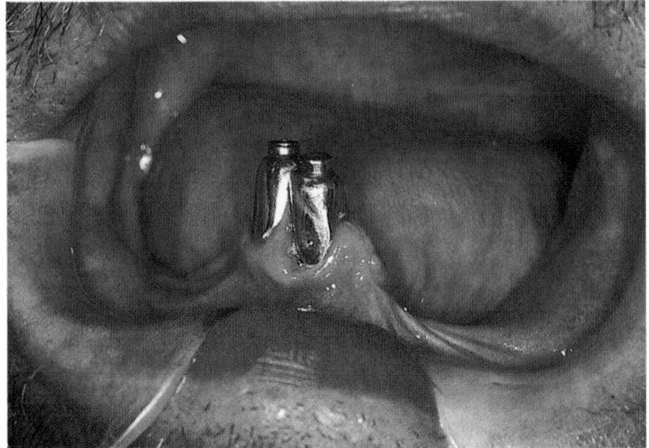

Fig. 4.25 Rothermann eccentric attachments.

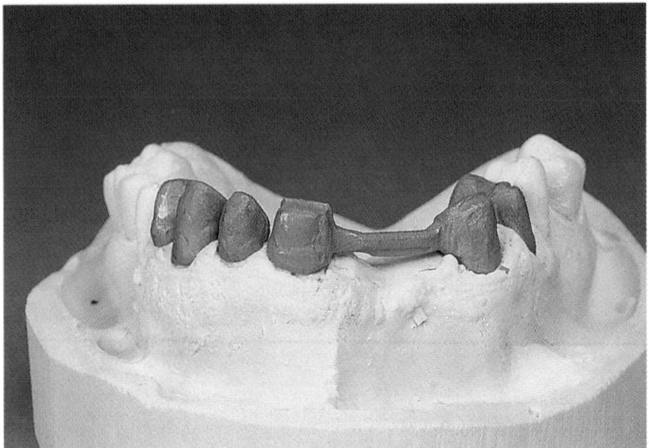

Fig. 4.27 Hader bar in a planned hybrid prosthesis.

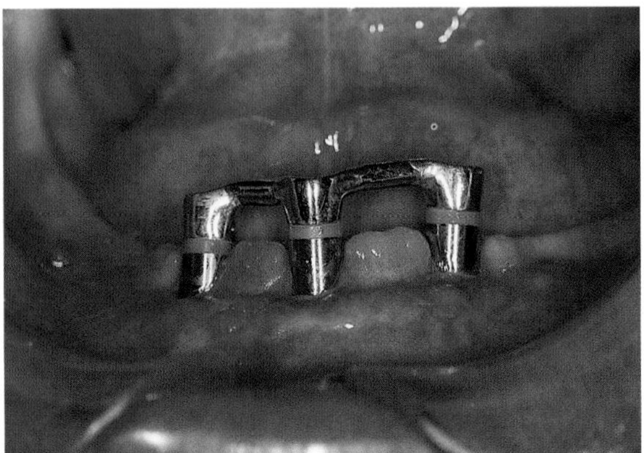

Fig. 4.26 Dolder bar.

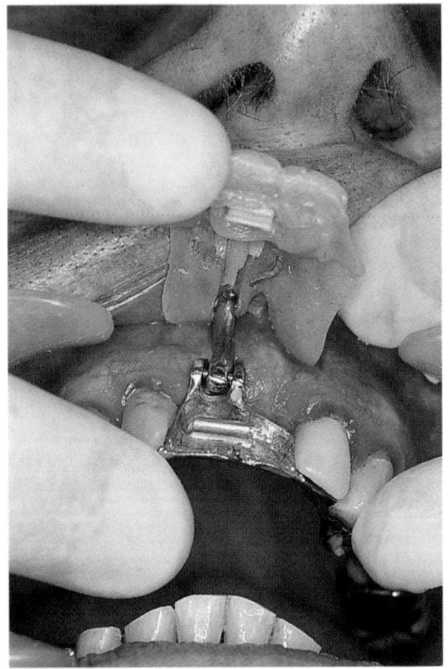

Fig. 4.28 Hinges in upper RPD.

Use of resilient materials

Two statements have already been made in this chapter which now need to be reviewed. The first was that, in theory, it is not possible to achieve a peripheral seal with a removable prosthesis. The second was the definition of a precision attachment (see above). Precision attachments are generally metallic, although some use polymeric components, e.g. rubber O-rings in stud attachments, and we offer the option of using traditional silicone rubber resilient base materials as retaining agents. Typical examples are where only two teeth remain in the arch. The patient is reluctant to lose the remaining teeth and the clinician may be apprehensive about extracting them. Conventional wisdom would indicate that the teeth may not have a lengthy prognosis and we offer the option of utilizing the remaining teeth and achieving a peripheral seal by enveloping them with a velum of silicone rubber (Fig. 4.36). This option is not suggested for every case, but only where the onset of edentulousness is perceived to be 2–3 years away. It must be pointed out to the patient that the resilient material will require to be replaced typically on an annual basis, much as the rubber component of the O-ring is.

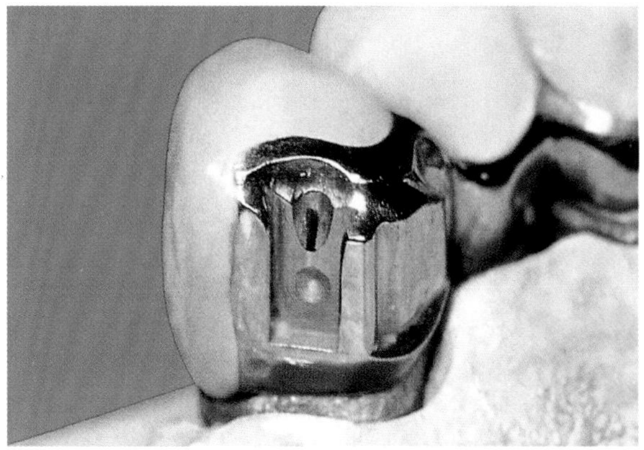

Fig. 4.29 A spring-leaded ball attachment would fit into this prepared receptacle in the matrix.

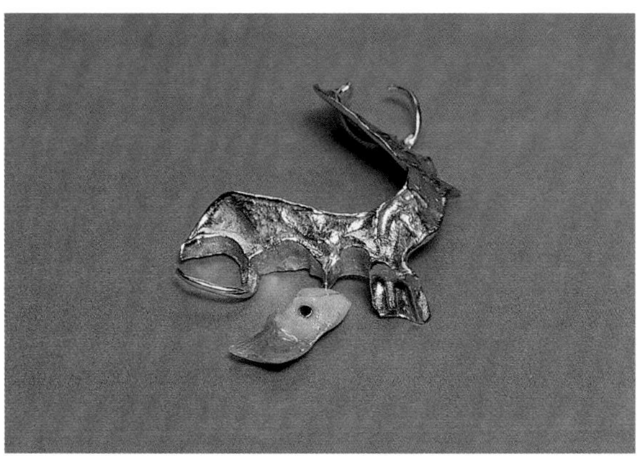

Fig. 4.30 Split-pin in tube. The tube is incorporated into the denture tooth.

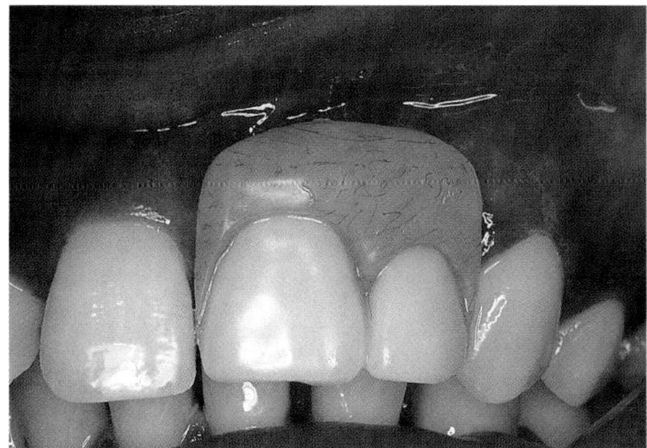

Fig. 4.31 Poor aesthetics, anterior saddle.

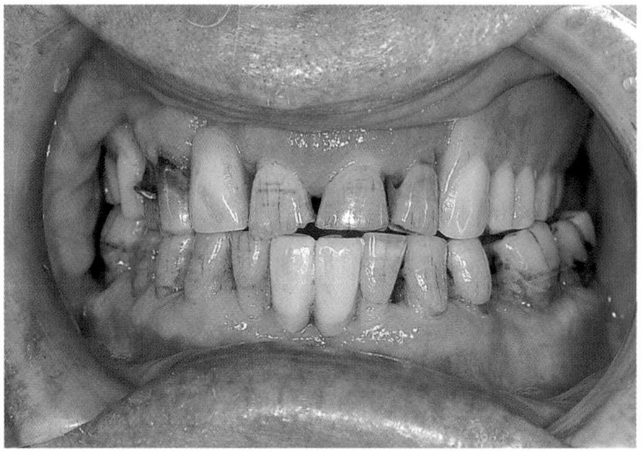

Fig. 4.32 Poor aesthetics, Kennedy I (modification).

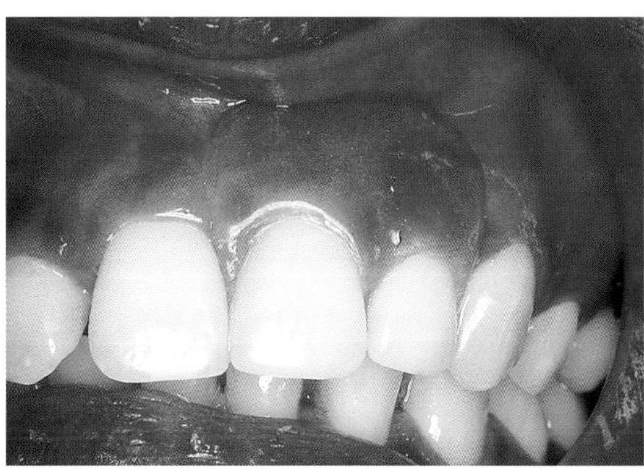

Fig. 4.33 Better result for Figure 4.31.

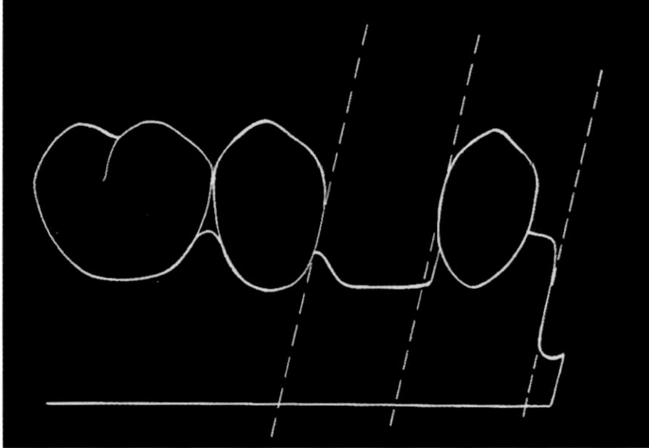

Fig. 4.34 The use of guide planes will improve retention and should enhance appearance.

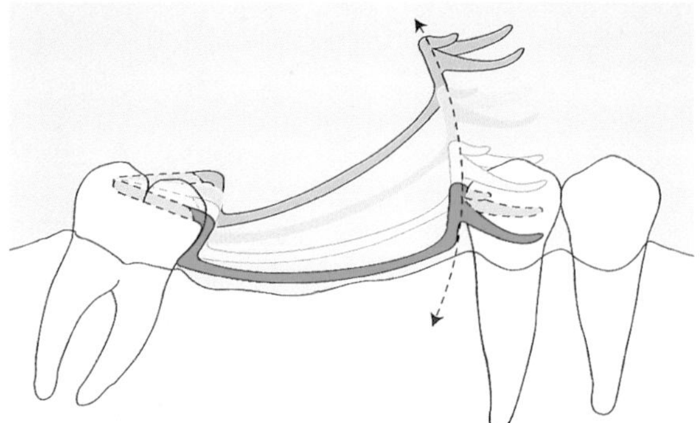

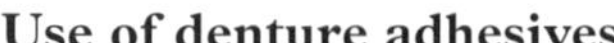

Fig. 4.35 Rotational path of insertion.

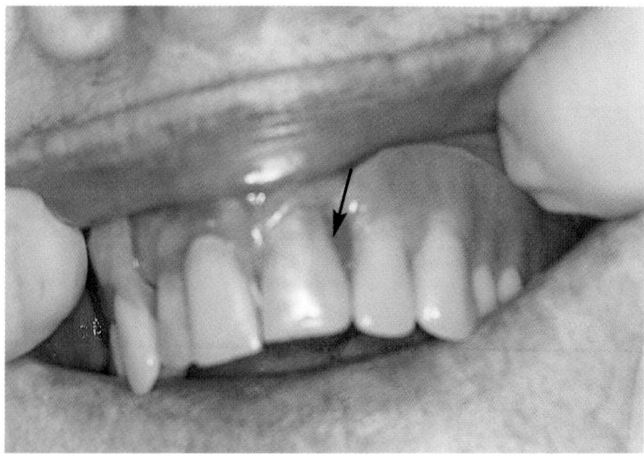

Fig. 4.36 Molloplast B has been added to engage the undercut on the distal of the abutment teeth (arrowed).

Use of denture adhesives

Most clinicians, if they are truthful, will confess that they have had to resort to recommending denture adhesives. This is typical in the case of complete dentures, as the potential for caries and other plaque-associated disease is enhanced if denture adhesives are worn in removable prostheses (Berg, 1991); nevertheless, patients will often resort to the use of denture adhesives if retention and stability are poor.

Planning for stability

If RPDs are to be worn with comfort and if they are to achieve their functional goals, then they ought to be as stable as possible during that function. Clearly, in mucosa-borne and in some tooth- and mucosa-borne RPDs, some fine movement of the denture bases over the saddle areas will occur. The principal area of concern is rotational movement. The element in an RPD that counteracts rotational movement is called **indirect retention,** and is achieved by one or more indirect retainers that reduce the tendency for a denture base to move in an occlusal direction about a fulcrum line.

An indirect retainer has been defined (Academy of Prosthodontics, 1999) as: 'the component of a removable partial denture that assists the direct retainer(s) in preventing displacement of the distal extension base by functioning through lever action on the opposite side of the fulcrum line when the denture base moves away from the tissues in pure rotation around the fulcrum line'.

The definition is not all-embracing, as indirect retainers may be incorporated in Kennedy IV dentures, where the saddle is, by definition, anteriorly placed.

The indirect retainer, in addition to resisting rotation of the saddle away from the tissues, also prevents the remainder of the denture, on the other side of the fulcrum, from traumatizing the tissues.

Some writers consider the fulcrum axis to be between the clasp tips; in the case of Kennedy 1 or 2 dentures (Kennedy, 1928), where the RPI system is used, this is essentially impossible and here the axis of rotation will be around the occlusal rests on the terminal abutment teeth (Fig. 4.37). In practice, the two axes tend to be so close to each other that the difference is of no practical significance.

It can be seen from Figure 4.37, therefore, that indirect retainers are supporting elements and serve to further stabilize the denture; failure to provide an indirect retainer will have the dual disadvantages of not resisting rotation and, by virtue of the rotation, will cause 'gum-stripping' by the denture.

Review of design with hygiene and maintenance in mind

After the clinician has drawn the design of the intended RPD on the study cast (Fig. 4.38) he/she

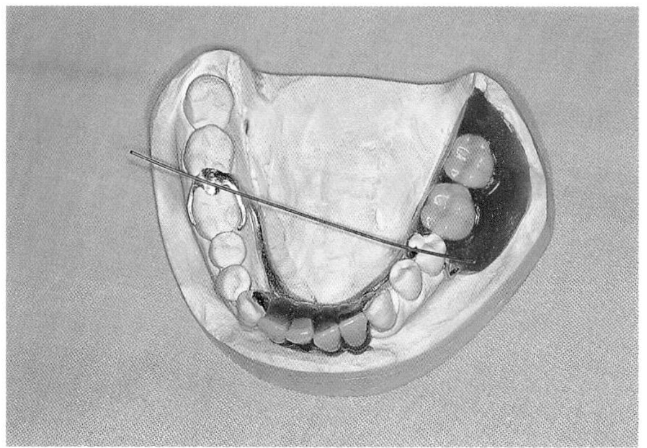

Fig. 4.37 The axis of rotation of this denture is indicated by the metal wire. This wire lies across the occlusal rests, and also coincides with the position of the clasp tip on the lower left premolar.

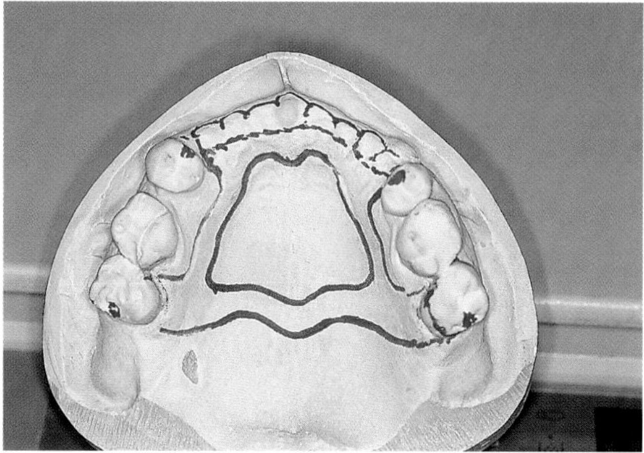

Fig. 4.38 Design drawn on cast.

should then review the design with an objective mind, to determine whether the RPD will be manageable by the patient, that it satisfies guidelines governing the health of tissues (e.g. 3 mm biological width or clearance from the free gingival margins), and that maintenance is relatively easy. For example, there is no point in designing an elaborate sectional denture if the patient does not have the dexterity to insert or remove it.

From the above, if the RPD is to be successful, then the clinician has a duty to plan removable prostheses appropriately for each patient. For this reason, the clinician should not abdicate responsibility by requesting the technician merely to make a prosthesis. No self-respecting clinician would prescribe a drug for a patient, without checking that it was appropriate to do so, yet many dentists request removable prostheses to be designed and processed by technicians who have never seen the patient and who have no real knowledge of the hard and soft dental tissues in the vicinity of the prostheses.

The simple template suggested in this chapter is recommended to enable the clinician to plan the most appropriate prosthesis for the patient.

REFERENCES

Academy of Prosthodontics. The glossary of prosthodontic terms, 7th edn. J Prosthet Dent 1999; 81: 39–110

Bates JF. The mechanical properties of the cobalt-chromium alloys and their relation to partial denture design. Br Dent J 1965; 119: 389–396

Bates JF, Neill DJ, Prieskel HW. Restoration of the partially dentate mouth. London: Quintessence Books, 1984

Beckett LS. The influence of saddle classification on the design of partial removable restorations. J Prosthet Dent 1953; 3: 506–516

Berg E. A clinical comparison of four denture adhesives. Int J Prosthodont 1991; 4: 449–456

Craddock FW. Prosthetic dentistry – a clinical outline, 3rd edn. London: Henry Kimpton, 1956

Kennedy E. Partial denture construction. New York: Dental Items of Interest Publishing Co, 1928

Kratochvil FJ. Influence of occlusal rest position and clasp design on movement of abutment teeth. J Prosthet Dent 1963; 13: 114–124

Krol AJ. Clasp design for extension base removable partial dentures. J Prosthet Dent 1973; 29: 408–415

Krol AJ, Finzen FC. Rotational path removable partial dentures. Part 1. Replacement of posterior teeth. Int J Prosthodont 1988; 1: 17–27

Kydd WL, Daly CH. The biologic and mechanical effects of stress on oral mucosa. J Prosthet Dent 1982; 47: 317–329

McCord JF, Smith GA, Quayle AA. Aesthetic provisional restoration the partially edentulous, immediate, postimplantation patient. Int J Prosthodont 1992; 5: 154–157

Osborne J, Lammie GA. Partial dentures, 4th edn. Oxford: Blackwell Scientific Publications, 1974

Picton DCA, Wills DJ. Viscoelastic properties of the periodontal ligament and mucous membrane. J Prosthet Dent 1978; 40: 263–272

Prabowa H. Applied technological aspects of cast cobalt chromium dental alloys. PhD thesis, University of Manchester, 1995
Preiskel HW. Precision attachments in dentistry, 3rd edn. London; Henry Kimpton, 1979
Wills DJ, Manderson RD. Biomechanical aspects of the support of partial dentures. J Dent 1977; 5: 310–318
Wills DJ, Manderson RD, Picton DCA. Biomechanics of the teeth and oral prostheses. In: Hastings GH, Williams DF, eds.) Mechanical properties of biomaterials. Bristol: J Wiley and Sons, 1980

5 Implant options

INTRODUCTION

The proven success of dental implants has, for suitable patients, revolutionized the prosthetic restoration of the dental arch following tooth loss and has significantly contributed to rehabilitation of the patient from a psychological and a functional perspective.

IMPLANT COMPONENTS/ OSSEOINTEGRATION

Dental implants, or more correctly the dental implant bodies, are usually of two forms, screw shaped or cylindrical, and are frequently made of commercially pure titanium (CPT). They function as analogues of tooth roots, achieving a union directly with jawbone following their insertion into a prepared 'socket' in the jaw. The process, which requires meticulous surgery and the avoidance of contamination of the implant surface, initially stabilizes the component either by its location against a threaded bony surface or by a wedged fit.

Contact between blood and the oxide film of the CPT implant body initiates the process of healing and bony repair that is associated with new bone growth. An established direct contact between the jawbone and the surface of the implant body ultimately permits the connection of the implant to a prosthesis that transmits occlusal forces directly to the jaw. This process is described as osseointegration and may be defined as: 'a process of clinically asymptomatic rigid fixation of alloplastic materials that is achieved and maintained in bone during functional loading'.

USES OF DENTAL IMPLANTS

Dental implants may stabilize a removable prosthesis (e.g. a complete or a partial overdenture) and/or support and stabilize a fixed prosthesis. There are three possibilities for the fixed restoration:

- Replacement of a single unit with a single tooth crown
- Replacement of several units using a fixed prosthesis supported by one or more implants (also referred to as an implant bridge)
- Replacement of the dental arch with a complete fixed prosthesis, again supported by several implants (this implant bridge may be a single unit, or several units which together restore the arch).

The potential prosthodontic options are:

- Fixed single tooth
- Fixed partial prosthesis
- Fixed complete prosthesis

- Removable partial overdenture
- Removable complete overdenture.

There are three major advantages of using dental implants:

- A stable removable prosthesis can eliminate most of the symptoms associated with the apparent or real looseness of conventional dentures. This tends to compromise a successful outcome to treatment for some patients. Stability arising from the attachment of the denture to the implant often eliminates pain, soreness, ulceration and retching.
- Fixed partial prostheses are confined to the local area of tooth loss, and so the risk of damage to other natural teeth and gingivae in contact with conventional dentures or following tooth preparation of abutment teeth is reduced or eliminated.
- Clearly, edentulous patients whose dentitions are restored by fixed prostheses supported by implants have the advantages associated with both of the former options, i.e. security of retention and limited coverage of the oral mucous membrane. This will have profound socio-psychological benefits.

IMPLANT COMPONENTS/RETENTION OF THE PROSTHESIS

Most implant systems have two components to which the prosthesis is secured. The dental implant body, lying in the jawbone, is intimately connected to an abutment which is secured most commonly by an abutment screw uniting the two. Various designs of linkage have been manufactured. Essentially the abutment may act as a female unit which fits on top of the implant body, for example the hexagonal-shaped projection from the implant, as in the Nobel Biocare system. Alternatively, it may be manufactured as a male unit forming an internal joint within the mouth of the implant, for example the so-called Morse taper projection linkage, as in the Astra Tech system (Binon, 2000).

Intrinsically there are three basic components:

- Dental implant body
- Abutment and abutment (screw) linkage
- Prosthesis and prosthetic linkage.

So that implant options may be considered comprehensively from the restorative dentistry point of view, their usage will be considered according to their design, namely fixed or removable.

Fixed restorative options

Here, the definitive (and perhaps the intermediate) prosthesis is either screwed to or cemented on to the abutment. When planning the case, this decision may be strongly influenced by the potential position of the access screw hole in the prosthesis. If it is foreseen that the artificial crown and implant are not in a straight alignment, then to avoid the access being in the labial face of the prosthetic crown it would be appropriate to cement on the unit. The aspects relevant to this consideration are:

- Cement or screw to abutment directly, e.g. single crown, fixed prosthesis
- Cement or screw component as part of prosthesis, e.g. cylinder within cast beam supporting dental arch of prosthesis.

When considering the design of a fixed prosthesis it is appropriate to ensure that the planned number of implants matches the extent of the occlusion to be restored in the arch and, further, that they are positioned optimally from both a functional and an aesthetic perspective.

A single unit requires a single implant to support it, but three units linked as a partial implant prosthesis may be supported by two implants. Although it is possible to use one implant and one natural tooth as 'bridge abutments', it is more common for the prosthesis to be supported by implants without linkage to natural teeth.

Manufacturers commonly provide components around which a crown or fixed prosthesis is constructed. For example, a gold alloy cylinder that can be screwed to the abutment can be part of a cast gold alloy beam carrying the teeth of the restored arch. In the case of a single crown, a ceramic cap can be provided to fit on to the abutment, and porcelain is fused to the cap to produce the crown that is ultimately cemented to the (titanium) abutment.

Removable restorative options

When designing removable prostheses two forms of anchorage are frequently used:

- A bar/sleeve (clip) joint where the bar links two or more implants
- A ball/cap anchorage applied individually to two or more isolated implants.

A third form of connection/anchorage may also be used, namely magnets/magnetic keepers, but these tend to afford less retention and are prone to corrosion (Davis, 1997).

In the case of sleeve retention, the bar is soldered to gold alloy cylinders which are screwed on to standard abutments; the sleeve is incorporated into the removable prosthesis and connects to the bar.

When prostheses obtain retention from ball anchorage, the balls are generally part of the abutment screws.

It should be pointed out that both types of anchorage require enough space within the denture to house the attachments in a sufficient volume of acrylic resin forming the base and body of the denture beneath the arch, so avoiding the risk of fracture: for this reason, it is important that wax trial dentures are viewed in situ and on the articulator to verify that appropriate space is present.

Anatomical considerations

Usually, a minimum of four implants linked by bars are inserted in the maxilla, whereas two are frequently used in the mandible in those areas of the edentulous arch normally associated with the canine and first premolar teeth. This is principally because the mandible has more cortical bone available for stability than the maxilla (Chan et al., 1998).

CHOOSING AN IMPLANT SOLUTION: MEETING THE GENERAL AND LOCAL CRITERIA

As was discussed in Chapters 1 and 2, a careful history and examination should enable the dentist to evaluate the treatment options and so weigh up the advantages of providing dental implants and the likelihood of their long-term success. There are certain aspects of the processes involved in these chapters that will be addressed in relation to implant considerations.

The patient's request for implant treatment should also be considered in the light of his/her understanding of the procedures and the length of this treatment, together with their previous experience of dentistry.

Implants can rarely recreate exactly the functions and appearance of the natural dentition, so that a dislike of conventional dentures or bridges and expectations that problems of retching and tolerance will be immediately solved by such devices are false hopes that should not be fostered. Implant treatment takes several months to complete. Likewise, implants ought not to be the automatic choice to replace failed conventional bridgework, for example because of insufficient bone, or poor standards of oral hygiene. A better understanding by the patient can of course, be achieved by discussion, the use of illustrative material, and by introducing one patient to another one who has successfully completed treatment. It is particularly important to be aware that a very small proportion of patients have emotional and psychiatric problems, including dysmorphophobic tendencies, and therefore that unrealistic expectations cannot be met by this complex care.

As was mentioned in Chapter 1, old age is not a contraindication when considering treatment (de Baat, 2000). However, it is wise to defer implant treatment in potential patients who have not reached dental maturity, for two reasons. First, participation in contact sports and similar activities may put the dentition at increased risk of traumatic damage and tooth loss. Secondly, implants in developing jaws may influence their relation with the prosthesis and between individual implants.

In addition, as most surgical procedures can be accomplished using local anaesthesia and sedation, the patient should be advised that general anaesthesia is only required for complex cases where there is difficulty of access, involvement of the facial skeleton, or where certain autogenous bone grafting procedures are required.

Other clinical considerations that should be particularly addressed relate to practical matters.

For example, three key features should be assessed during the information gathering sessions:

- The movement of the jaws and the gape for access to the arch and edentulous spans must allow appropriate instrumentation during the surgical and prosthetic procedures, in order to avoid malpositioning of implants or risks in handling components, e.g. abutments and prosthesis fixing screws etc., that could be dislodged into the airway.
- The intermaxillary relationships and associated occlusion may have a profound effect on positioning implants and positioning of the dental arch. A Class III jaw relation and a Class II relation associated with a Class II div 2 malocclusion tend to be difficult to manage.
- The characteristic behaviour of the lips may demonstrate excessive circumoral contraction or elevation/depression of the upper or lower lip during smiling and speaking. When the tooth crowns and alveolus are revealed ('high smile line') the design of the prostheses is critical. For example, partial restoration of the arch may be unaesthetic if the effect of alveolar resorption has not been considered, unless some form of bone augmentation is carried out. The artificial tooth/teeth may be excessive in length, a flange may be required, or the implant abutment may be revealed.
- Furthermore, lip contraction in the edentulous patient with an atrophied mandible may destabilize a lower implant-retained complete overdenture because of the dentist's failure to consider the available denture space in which the base and arch are to be sited. Indeed, without an appropriate surgical guide (stent) the implants themselves may be positioned too far labially or lingually, encroaching on the movement of the investing tissues.

Both clinical and radiological examination should reveal a good volume of good-quality bone to stabilize the implant in an appropriate relationship to the intended arch. Higher success rates of implant integration have been demonstrated over long periods of loading where long implants have been secured in bone. A rounded alveolar ridge with miminal resorption is likely to produce an effective anchorage. Similarly, immediate insertion into a healthy tooth socket, with further extension of the prepared bony canal to reach cortical bone, can provide the optimum anchorage. In such circumstances, standard implants of almost 4 mm diameter with lengths of 13–20 mm may be inserted. In the edentulous mandible the adverse features of a flat ridge may, on palpation, reveal a sufficient depth and width to the anterior aspect of the jaw to provide for the integration of five or six implants to retain a fixed cantilevered complete prosthesis.

Importantly, the radiographs should reveal the proximity of any conflicting structures. The location of the maxillary antrum, the incisive canal and the mandibular canal with mental orifice may inhibit the use of dental implants or restict their length.

In partially dentate subjects, consideration of the width of the span to be restored will help to decide on the number and position of implants to be placed to support the prosthesis. Careful planning must confirm adequate clearance between the adjacent natural tooth's periodontal membrane and the implant, which should ideally be positioned appropriately below the artificial tooth crown of the prosthesis. It is critical to compare the direction of the adjacent natural tooth crown with its root, apparent especially in the radiograph, and so avoid damage to the natural root from incorrect preparation of the bony canal that receives the implant.

Overerupted opposing natural teeth, or the presence of a deep overbite, may prevent the use of implants, as there may be insufficient space between the head of the implant set in the cortical layer of the jaw surface and the opposing teeth. There may be insufficient clearance even to allow the use of a minimum height of abutment.

Tables 5.1, 2 and 3 give general and specific considerations for implant therapy.

ADVANTAGES OF TREATMENT WITH DENTAL IMPLANTS

Patients considered suitable for dental implants as a result of a satisfactory history and examination gain various advantages from treatment, depending on the design of the prosthesis. However, all

Table 5.1 Adverse factors contraindicating/ inhibiting implant treatment

General factors	Local factors
Severe physical/mental illness, e.g. frail elderly; Alzheimer's disease, psychiatric illness/depression Active malignancy Specific medical conditions, e.g. uncontrolled diabetes, cardiovascular disease (bleeding tendency/stroke, subacute bacterial endocarditis risk) Substance abuse, e.g. tobacco (heavy smoker), alcohol, narcotics etc. Unrealistic expectations, e.g. dysmorphobia	Recurrent caries, uncontrolled periodontal disease in dentition Extensively restored dentitions with dubious prognosis Poor quality/quantitiy of bone Limited space for components, e.g. reduced span, deep overbite Unfavourable jaw relations, e.g. Class III, Class II Restricted gape

Table 5.2 Potential alternative treatments

Option	Restorative option
Single unit	Single tooth implant Conventional bridge Resin-bonded bridge Partial denture (RPD)
Multiple units in single arch span	Fixed implant partial prosthesis Conventional bridge Resin-bonded bridge RPD with/without overdenture, natural tooth abutments
Complete arch replacement	Fixed complete implant prosthesis Removable complete implant overdenture prosthesis Conventional denture or overdenture prosthesis
Complex restorations	Crowns and bridges and implant restorations (fixed and removable) Crowns and bridges and partial dentures (RPDs)

Table 5.3 Factors to consider when treating a partially dentate patient with implants

Categories	Factors
General patient factors	Is it likely that there will be further tooth loss? Will further tooth loss compromise treatment?
General dental/ oral factors	Does the span need restoration? Is the remaining dentition healthy? Is there adequate quantity/quality of bone? Can sufficient implants be sited appropriately?
General restorative	Is there adequate space for the implant superstructure? Will the appearance and function be optimal? Is there a risk of damage (trauma, parafunction)?

gain the benefit of the local retention of bone at the sites for implantation, rather than experiencing the unpredictable effects of alveolar resorption. Where bone is not subject to adverse loading from the implant restoration, healing and remodelling in the first year may result in a horizontal reduction of 1–2 mm at the head of the implant, and less than 0.2 mm annually may be expected in successful cases of implantation using a threaded titanium analogue (Adell et al., 1981). This represents a substantial benefit over conventional treatment.

A major advantage over conventional fixed options is that single units restoring a span for one tooth require no other preparation of adjacent natural teeth, especially those with virgin surfaces. This frequently arises in younger adults with minimal or no caries experience. In addition, where longer spans exist and where the adjacent natural teeth are inappropriate for consideration as bridge abutments (because of their morphology, e.g. short crown, small root area etc.), these spans can be usefully restored with fixed implant-borne prostheses.

Dental implants offer advantages in specific situations that are either impractical or poorly managed by conventional bridges or dentures. Both long bounded saddles and distal extension spans may be treated when several implants can restore tooth loss, provided appropriate loading can be achieved.

Clearly, dental implants are not subject to root caries and so patients restored with an implant-borne removable prosthesis may be spared the potential for loss of natural teeth in contact with a conventional denture. Hence, when some terminal dentitions are restored it may be more appropriate to provide dental implants to stabilize a denture or a fixed bridge, thereby avoiding the traditional use of tooth abutments. For example, lower natural canine teeth replaced by dental implants may prove a more durable, cost-effective solution when constructing a complete overdenture.

As the loss of teeth is inevitably followed by alveolar resorption and, further, as dental implants have the capacity to inhibit alveolar ridge reduction following extractions, then 'priority' treatment has been suggested. These situations occur where patients with some 40 or more years of life expectancy have become edentulous (or will soon be rendered so) in one or both jaws. Congenital and acquired deficiencies of the jaws may also warrant implant treatment, for example if patients have hypodontia, where their dentition is compromised as a result of a hereditary defect.

The construction of a prosthesis following jaw resection is a challenge both for the dentist and for the patient, who has to wear the appliance. The use of implants following autogenous grafting and/or soft tissue revision permits the construction of a stable prosthesis.

An aesthetic improvement can be achieved for partially dentate patients, especially when the alveolar ridge and mucosal coverage have an optimum morphology. The emergence profile of single units and the form of pontics may achieve a close resemblance to natural teeth. Any display of clasps used to retain partial dentures, or alloy from bridge units, or the retentive 'wings' of resin-bonded bridges is eliminated. Careful case analysis is always required, and where a less than ideal aesthetic outcome is predicted, although some benefits will be envisaged, detailed discussion of the planned result with the patient will be essential.

The summation of all of the planning has to be the satisfaction that certain functional and aesthetic criteria are met. These considerations may be summarized as follows:

- Will the implants be located appropriately below the individual artificial teeth in the prosthesis?
- Will the labial mucosa be evident?
- Will the artificial tooth crown(s) be positioned abnormally?
- Will the crowns appear longer than the adjacent natural teeth?
- Will the titanium abutment be visible?
- Will a flange be required, and will the border be obvious?

These considerations are listed in Table 5.4.

The importance of considering implant therapy holistically cannot be emphasized too strongly, and the planning, insertion and restoration of the implants, plus long-term maintenance, should be seen as one. For simplicity, however, the surgical and prosthodontic options will be considered under separate headings.

Surgical considerations

A successful outcome of implant treatment is dependent on careful surgical and prosthetic assessment, followed by planned procedures to achieve the desired result. When evaluating the evidence, the dental surgeon will have considered seven essential aspects beyond the general considerations of suitability for a surgical procedure. These are:

- Is there sufficient volume of bone to house the implants?
- Will bony defects created by resorption or the natural jaw shape limit the position and direction of the implant?

Table 5.4 Considerations for and advantages of implant-supported prostheses in an edentulous jaw

Considerations	Advantages
Has the patient tolerated/successfully worn a conventional, well designed prosthesis? Is the opposing jaw dentate, or edentulous with atrophic tissues? Is there sufficient volume of bone to include 4–6 implants, or 2–3 implants? Will resorption dictate using a flange? Will bony augmentation be required? Will positions of the implants be compatible with the position of the dental arch? Is the jaw relation favourable, with space for components, producing good arch alignment?	Stable reconstruction. For a fixed bridge, (eliminating movement in function; for complete overdentures, reducing movement in function) Less mucosal coverage than a RPD. This is unlikely to apply to an overdenture stabilized by two implants, where full mucosal coverage will be necessary to provide adequate stability Better tolerance Less impairment of masticatory function

- Will any dehiscences be manageable using a membrane, or should the jaw be augmented before implantation (Triplett et al., 2000)?
- Will the number and position of implants be restricted by vital structures?
- Is there sufficient access to the span, and will the implant be capable of being orientated suitably in relation to the natural teeth, other implants and the intended prosthesis?
- Will the implants emerge at an appropriate site?
- Will the surgery improve or affect the aesthetic outcome, especially when soft tissues contours around the restoration should resemble gingivae?

The outcome of this evaluation must be shared by members of the specialist team if the dental surgeon himself is not carrying through both surgical and prosthodontic treatments.

Guide to implant placement

Having decided on the expected number and size(s) of implants to be used, and having considered the likely abutments needed to support the restoration, a surgical template must be prepared to assist the surgeon at the time of implantations. The template (surgeon's guide or stent) is prepared from a trial denture or diagnostic wax-up prepared on the articulated study casts, and it may be a modified facsimile of a prosthesis processed in PMMA or it may be made of another polymer, e.g. PVA. The design should permit the surgeon to position it on the teeth adjacent to the site, or, in edentulous jaws, on the ridges remote from the area for drilling the bony canals (Figs 5.1a & b).

Some operators prefer a channel to guide the direction of the bur penetrating the bone after the flap is raised. Others choose to have the occlusal and labial face only represented, so that access and angulation can be adjusted behind the line of the arch and the particular artificial teeth in the span. The guide must not impede vertical movement of the bur/drill, and in narrow spans for single tooth replacement, drill extensions or long-shanked components are required.

Flap design and operative principles

The design of the flap must provide good access to the width of the jaw surface, and in partially dentate arches it is crucial to decide whether sulcar incisions around the adjacent teeth, or those that preserve the gingival cuffs of the adjacent teeth, are to be used. This is to avoid recessions around the teeth adjacent to the span.

An appropriate surgical protocol is used that prepares the canal and inserts the correct length of implant so that the implant head lies at or just below the superior surface of the bony cortical plate. A series of twist or spade drills are used to create and enlarge the canal under a constant flow of cool saline, in order to maintain a temperature below 47°C and avoid overheating the bone.

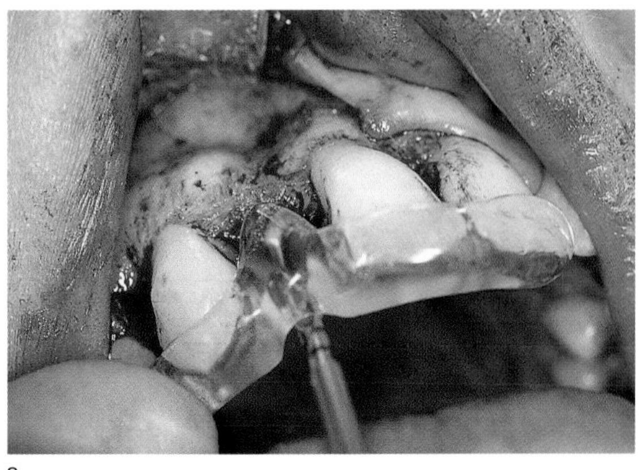
a

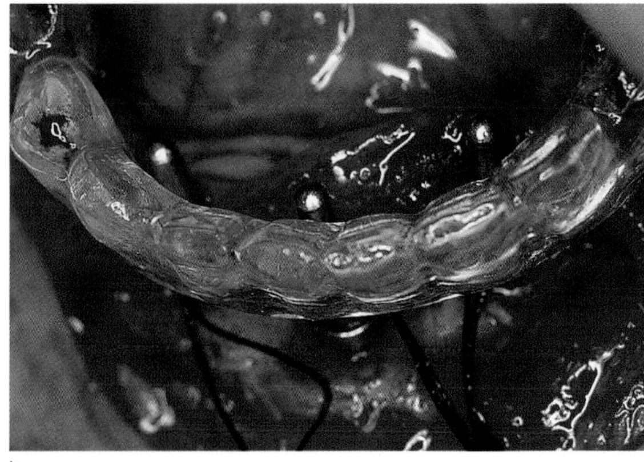
b

Fig. 5.1 Positioning the surgical template to ensure appropriate alignment of the dental implant with the intended restored arch in (a) a partially dentate jaw and (b) an edentulous jaw. Note that the bony canals prepared by drills can be verified with direction indicators before the implant is positioned.

At operation, the surgeon has a choice of implants with varying diameters and lengths. Most commonly a standard-diameter threaded implant long enough to engage an optimum depth of bone is used. If it is foreseen or appreciated at operation that the direction of the implant within the jaw is at variance with the orientation of the future artificial crown, it is helpful if an angulated guide (direction indicator) can be placed in the canal to judge to what depth the implant should be positioned in order to subsequently carry a suitable angulated abutment.

The surgeon should not hope that the prosthodontist will be able to utilize a poorly positioned implant by selecting/creating an abutment to overcome a problem of misalignment: this is very rarely possible to achieve.

To ensure that implants are correctly spaced to support partial or complete fixed prostheses it is helpful for the surgeon to have the preoperative study casts marked by the dentist to show the preferred location of each one. Implants do not have to be positioned in a straight line, although such positioning creates a straight fulcrum axis about the support. For edentulous subjects, implants lie in a curved arrangement, usually anterior to the antra and mental nerve foraminae in the jaws. In spans of the partially dentate jaw, slight convergence of the implant heads from the vertical axis creates better resistance to lateral loading, while lying in the curve of the arch within the jaw.

It is desirable to avoid loading the implant immediately, and so most patients are advised that implants should remain buried for 3 months in the mandible and 6 months in the maxilla to optimise osseointegration. Usually 2 weeks is required after implantation to permit good soft tissue wound healing before a transitional denture is inserted. A temporary resin-bonded bridge may be placed for short spans.

At the second surgical stage to expose the implant head and remove the cover screw a healing abutment is placed through the mucosa. If a small flap is raised the patient will have been warned about a further healing period of 7–10 days before the temporary prostheses can be repositioned. However, some systems employ a single surgical stage in which a component penetrates the mucosa immediately.

PROSTHODONTIC TREATMENT CONSIDERATIONS

Although preoperative planning may anticipate the likely design of the prosthesis, in many cases the particular issues about the final choice of abutments cannot be resolved until an impression is recorded that relates the exact position of each implant head to the edentulous jaw and the arch of natural teeth.

This is achieved with a special tray and a suitable impressions material (e.g. a polyether such as Impregum) that records transfer impression copings located on the implant heads and temporarily secured with fixing screws (Figs. 5.2a & b). Patients must be advised preoperatively that an intraoral radiograph may be required to confirm their correct seating when the healed cuff margin is superficial to a deeply placed implant head.

The master impression is poured in dental stone and should be modified with a silicone insert to represent the mucosal cuffs (Fig. 5.3). This enables the emergence profile of the implant body and/or abutment to be expanded by a prosthesis when the abutment shoulder is 'subgingival'.

The cast contains dummy replica fixtures which are screwed to the impression copings before the impression is cast.

At this stage it is possible for the dental surgeon and the dental technician to agree upon the choice of a suitable abutment. This may be an exact precision shape available from the manufacturer, or one that is created by scanning the cast with and without a custom-built wax/resin replica, which enables an individual milled abutment to be produced in the laboratory (Brunton et al., 1999).

Manufacturers provide 'dummy abutments' which are tried on the replica implant head so that the angle, shoulder depth and prosthetic connection can be optimized (Figs 5.4, 5.5).

The dental surgeon will have initially agreed with the patient whether an acrylic resin/gold alloy frame or a porcelain/alloy prosthesis will be chosen. Usually a reduction in the alveolus requires the former to restore the missing tissue form in fixed prostheses. For a removable prosthesis, the choice between a bar/sleeve (clip) or ball/cap anchorage should have already been made.

If it is clear on applying a dental index of the future arch against the master cast that there is limited space which restricts the volume of acrylic resin over the implants, then a cast metal strengthener must be incorporated in the overdenture design; otherwise, there is a risk of fatigue failure of the prosthesis. It should not be forgotten that such retaining devices require the technician to 'block out' undercuts to allow caps and sleeves to expand, and for interferences around

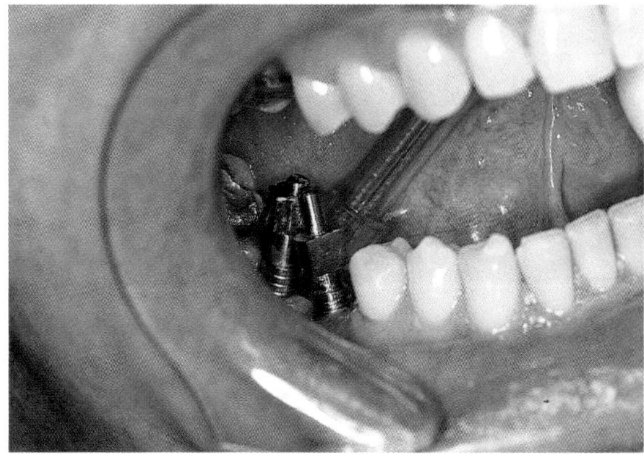

a

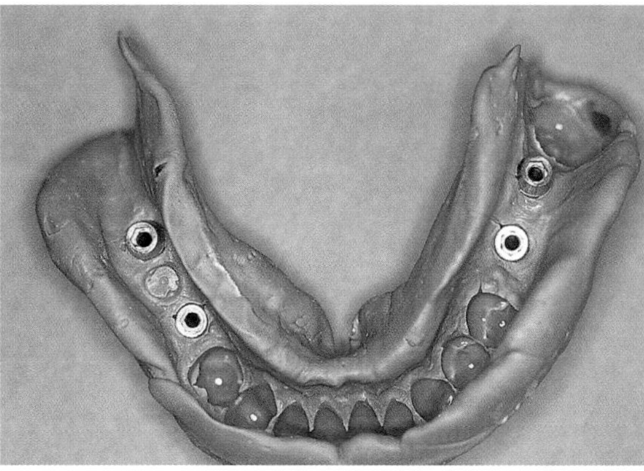

b

Fig. 5.2 (a) Transfer impression copings secured to the top of the dental implant body and (b) located in an impression recorded in a special tray, for a partially dentate jaw.

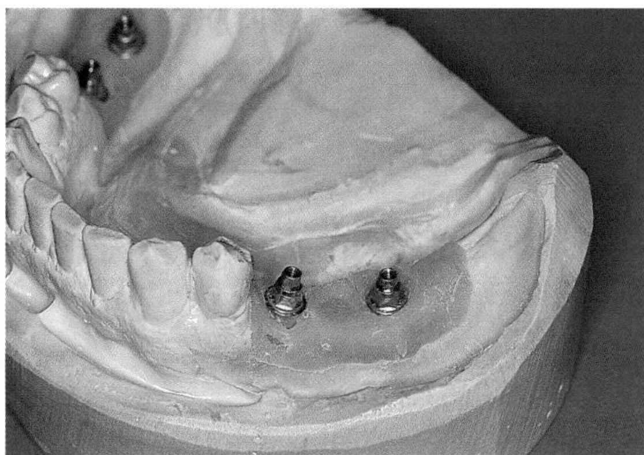

Fig. 5.3 Master cast poured from a partially edentulous jaw, including a silicone cuff surrounding the implant heads, represented by replicas with two chosen abutments in position.

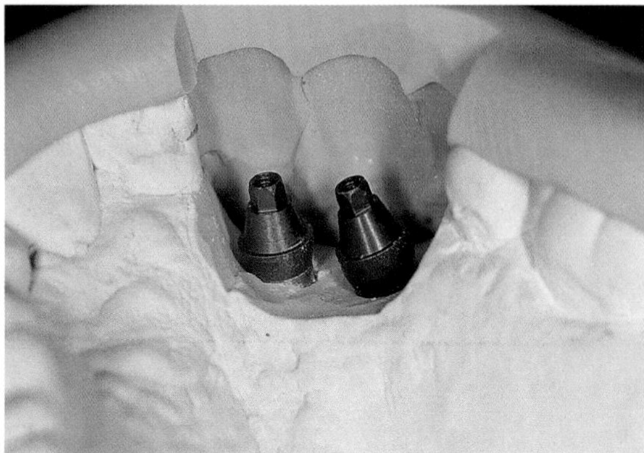

Fig. 5.4 Dummy abutments, selected in the laboratory and positioned in the cast with the appropriate collar depth and angulation.

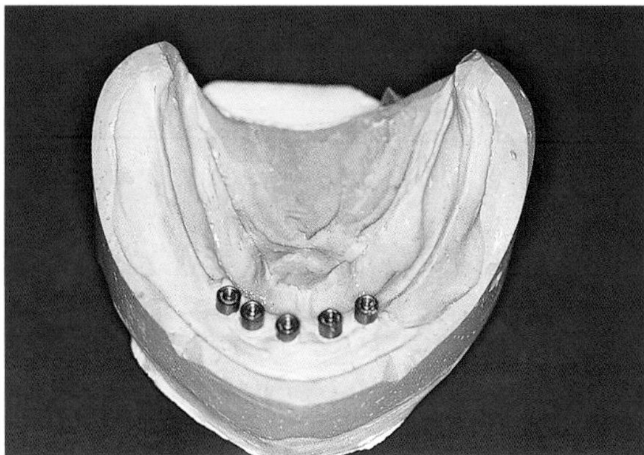

Fig. 5.5 Master cast poured from an edentulous jaw enclosing replica standard abutments.

abutments to be eliminated in order to insert overdentures.

Examples of the laboratory and clinical procedures to be followed are available in texts and information from the manufacturers (Hobkirk & Watson, 1995). Such illustrative material is helpful in explaining the treatment plan. Catalogues of components supplied by manufacturers are essential for planning because of the variety of components. Each has variable dimensions, so that its precise position in relation to the implant head and the restored arch can be assessed.

Forethought must be given to the design of the occlusion. Obviously the prosthesis should form part of a balanced occlusion. Where there is evidence that the patient may clench or grind teeth, the restored partially dentate arch should be protected by a removable soft bite guard worn during sleep. Similarly, the retentive elements, e.g. bar anchorage, can be protected when complete or partial overdentures are removed at night. Both single crowns and partial fixed prostheses are vulnerable to loosening of the abutment screws or prosthesis fixing screws if eccentric interferences exist. In addition, artificial teeth in overdentures and fixed prostheses are susceptible to wear or fracture. Patients should be warned of this possibility and the consequent need for regular monitoring (Table 5.5).

Table 5.5 Ideal outcome of implant restoration

Factor	Requirement
Good patient cooperation	Maintaining excellent oral hygiene Avoiding excessive loading of implant – e.g. bruxism Producing normal loading – avoiding trauma Regular review of dental health
Sustained integration of implants	Non-mobility of each implant Less than 0.2 mm annual bone loss (after year 1) Asymptomatic No inflammation of mucosal cuff
Successful restoration	Secure cement or screw retention Sustained occlusion without abnormal wear Aesthetic with mucosal/ alveolar contours maintained

FOLLOW-UP AND MAINTENANCE OUTCOMES

During the planning stage, when the patient is, or ought to be, informed of treatment options and outcomes, they should also be informed that osseointegration is a biomechanical process and that therefore there are specific survival rates for both the implant and the prosthesis, which are influenced by both the patient and the design/treatment.

Implant failure/survival

At worst, the implant may fail early, and because of a 'cluster effect' all implants can fail to integrate in a patient. This unfavourable host response to integration is more common in those who have a poor quality/quantity of bone, and where adverse general conditions exist, e.g. smoking, radiotherapy.

Short-term failure, e.g. usually within 2 years of loading, may be precipitated by adverse forces applied to the prosthesis. Those patients who exhibit bruxism can experience this problem. Likewise, a poorly fitting prosthesis screwed to a 'tight misfit' against the abutment, or excessive buccal/labial or mesiodistal cantilevering, may induce bone loss.

Marginal bone loss arising from adverse forces, especially when coincident with inflammation of the mucosal cuff as an established 'perimplantitis', may produce 'cratering'. This renders the implant liable to fatigue failure, usually at the level of the apical end of the abutment screw. There are two possible indicators of implant failure. First, the implant site may be mildly painful, and when the prosthesis is removed the implant is found to be mobile and easily unwound from the bone. Secondly, the implant may fracture and be unsuitable for modification, so that the only course will be to trephine the fractured component from the bone, which is then allowed to heal before further evaluation.

Fortunately, with an experienced operator and a well motivated patient such severe problems are uncommon. The dentist should, of course, be aware of evidence-based cumulative survival rates published by expert centres (Adell et al., 1981; Cooper et al., 1999; Lekholm et al., 1999; Priest, 1999).

Monitoring

Monitoring is conducted at regular intervals, more frequently early on after the completion of inserting and loading the implant, in order to ensure that the patient is pain free and functioning efficiently, as well as personally maintaining high standards of oral hygiene around the prosthesis and abutments.

The dentist will also be responsible for:

- Testing the security of the prosthesis and abutment screws
- Checking that cemented structures remain luted in position
- Monitoring the RPD implant – stabilized prosthesis, particularly the retaining sleeves, clips or caps, as well as conventional maintenance to the denture
- Monitoring the opposing arch, e.g. in edentulous patients a conventional denture opposing the implanted jaw may also need careful supervision to avoid loss of retention or the effects of imbalance in the occlusion, as a result of resorption of the opposing ridge. A list of the requirements for maintenance is listed in Table 5.6.

It is highly desirable to encourage patients to attend immediately problems arise, however simple, so that unforeseen major repairs are avoided and the patient does not face an 'unexpected disaster', with loss of confidence in the treatment.

It is, however, inevitable that the dentist will need to remove the prosthesis to renew components, e.g. a fractured fixing prosthesis screw or retentive clip (Watson & Davis, 1996). Any interim prosthesis and healing caps used to cover abutments should be retained for such an eventuality.

Planning aftercare

Aftercare may involve resolving peri-implant mucosal health or mechanical problems associated with:

- The prosthesis
- The abutment, with its linkages either to the implant or to the prosthesis.

This is achieved via:

- Correcting the patient's hygiene methods: scaling abutments; removal of prosthesis for cleaning

Table 5.6 Routine monitoring requirements

Requirement	Objective
Examination of mucosa	Confirming absence of per-abutment inflammation, mucosal sinus, traumatic ulceration
Examination of implant with long cone 'periapical' radiograph	Excludes horizontal bone loss, loss of contact with implant
Detachment of prosthesis	To confirm secure abutment, immobility of implant
Examination of prosthesis	To confirm fixed prosthesis is immobile Absence of facets of wear on occlusal surfaces of teeth Occlusion is balanced, screw access is sealed Anchorage effective for overdentures

- Securing retention mechanisms: adjusting retentive clips, caps for overdenture; tightening prosthesis fixing screws; removing prosthesis to tighten abutment screw
- Adjustment to occlusion: eliminating eccentric interferences/wear facets; remounting prosthesis on articulator (complete/partial overdenture).

The health of the mucosal cuff is dependent on good access and effective cleaning. Many patients will require regular specific hygiene training and monitoring to produce low plaque and calculus levels. Where problems are foreseen, it is appropriate to establish a regular programme before implantation is attempted.

In patients for whom overdentures using bar retention is planned, the bar should be effectively spaced from the mucosa and planning should be directed to instructing the patient in brushing and flossing both the inferior bar surface and the opposing mucosa. For those with fixed prostheses the use of 'supa-floss' and 'proxy brushes' of a suitable diameter should be taught (Fig. 5.6).

Trauma to the oral mucosa from the denture, attributable to minor faults in the extension of the base or occlusion, should be anticipated in cases of gross atrophy, so that the normal corrective procedures, including remounting the prosthesis on an articulator, are expected.

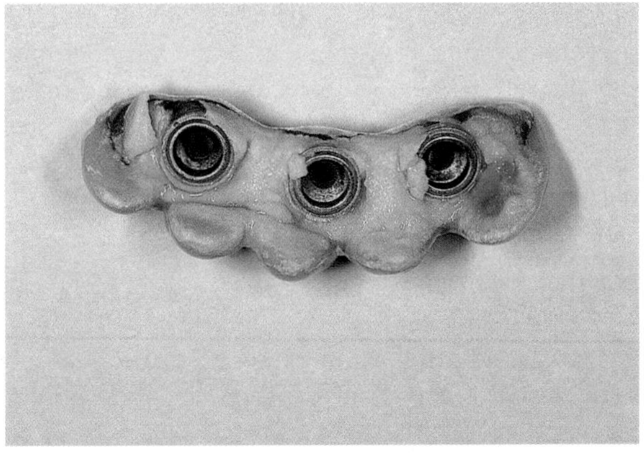

Fig. 5.6 Use of a suitable size and shape of proxy brush will remove plaque from beneath the prosthesis around the abutments. The accumulated debris can clearly be seen on the removed bridge's impression surface.

The avoidance of mechanical problems

Looseness of either the abutment screw or the prosthesis fixing screw is more frequent when there is instability of an overdenture, or leverage as a result of the cantilevering of a fixed prosthesis so that the preload sustaining intimate contact of abutment and implant is exceeded. The dentist must therefore select implants of the optimum diameter and tighten to a predetermined torque level to optimize tension in the screw, so as to prevent the joint opening. Wider diameter implants, e.g. 5 or 6 mm rather than 3.75 mm diameter standard ones, have a broader surface area to the implant platform and screws of greater diameter. These are an appropriate choice in the molar area, where there is sufficient jaw width to resist the larger occlusal loading that may affect standard implants and abutments.

Problems of looseness of the abutment screw associated with single implant prostheses are now overcome in some systems by using gold alloy screws inserted with a higher torque (32N cm as opposed to 20N cm) (Jorneus et al., 1992).

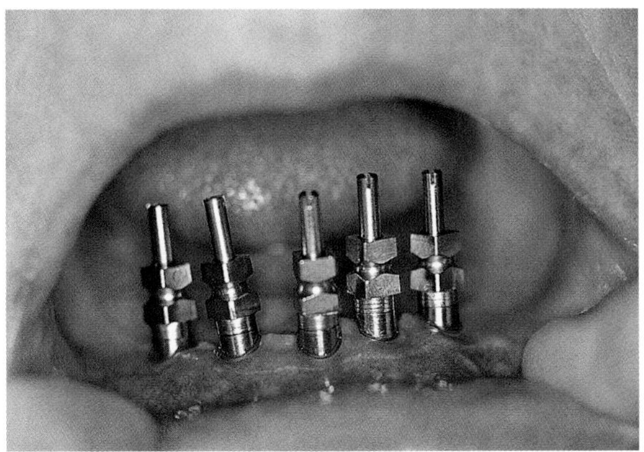

Fig. 5.7 These abutments have been positioned in the mouth on the dental implants before the impression is made using abutment transfer impression copings.

When planning to use narrow platform implants of 3.2 mm diameter, for example, it is important to appreciate that the location of the abutment may be more difficult, e.g. CeraOne (Fig. 5.7).

Looseness may reflect either an inexact fit (Fig. 5.8) or an eccentric occlusal interference, so that contacts with the opposing arch create screw looseness, or, alternatively, decementation of the crown. Patients should be warned that a crown can decement and that they should push it back into position and avoid removing it, so that the mucosal cuff does not collapse or the mucosa heal over the head of the implant, and return for consultation as soon as possible.

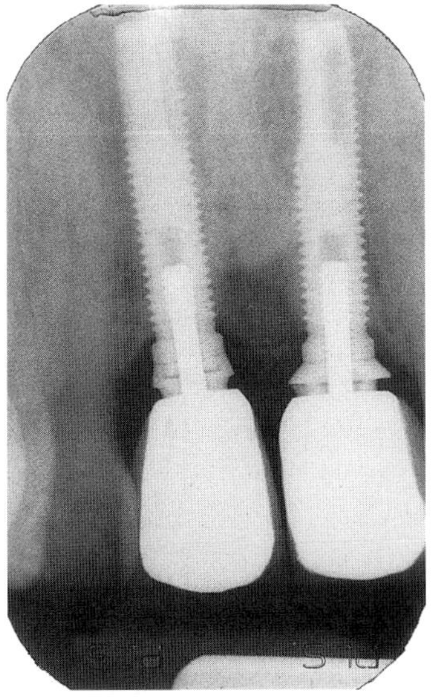

Fig. 5.8 Radiograph showing the failure to seat crowns on components.

Fatigue failure

In some patients fatigue failure of a cantilever beam can occur, especially where:

- The opposing arch and level of occlusal plane has resulted in the framework having to be reduced in bulk because of lack of space
- An overoptimistic extension of the cantilever beyond 10–13 mm has been used to increase the length of the occlusal table opposing natural teeth.

DESIGNING THE OCCLUSION TO AVOID PROSTHETIC PROBLEMS

Careful consideration must be given to the design of the occlusion. Where resin teeth are used in an acrylic resin/gold alloy-framed prosthesis it is important to be aware that occlusal forces, especially those associated with parafunction, will abrade the teeth and unbalance the occlusion (Lang & Razzoog, 1992; Denissen et al., 1993). In fixed prostheses artificial teeth may fracture or detach from the resin, whereas in removable implant prostheses symptoms of soreness and pain associated with trauma from the base may arise.

It is particularly crucial to assess the natural occlusion in eccentric jaw relations and detect facets of tooth wear. When a fixed prosthesis is planned, bonded ceramic structures should harmonize with the existing natural occlusion. Premature occlusal contacts on the implant-supported prosthesis may:

- Loosen the screw retainers
- Decement the prosthesis (e.g. single crown)
- Fracture the porcelain.

Unforeseen maintenance can be costly, and occasionally damage is not easily rectified without remaking the prosthesis.

Creating a pleasing appearance

Avoiding complaints of an unsatisfactory appearance is an essential part of planning treatment, especially where the arch and alveolus are evident during smiling and speech. Hence, it must be made clear whether part or all of the artificial tooth crowns will be revealed, and if the gingival anatomy or the components, such as abutments, will be evident.

Obviously a low smile-line is much less likely to give rise to complaints than when the alveolar mucosa is displayed, as only part of the prosthesis is evident. However, it is important when planning treatment to use photographs to discuss the issues that may produce a less than ideal outcome, and the possible options that exist to avoid difficulties.

A diagnostic wax-up for a single crown or partial fixed prosthesis may be required during treatment. If a trial tooth arrangement is inserted for the patient's inspection before surgical treatment, it is essential to set the teeth in a manner similar to the expected outcome, i.e. gum fitted rather than with a flange.

Following extraction of the natural tooth the alveolar volume reduces, so that it is not uncommon for the implant to support a crown longer than the adjacent natural teeth. If there is likely to be a clear disparity in size a choice must be made. The clinician must therefore decide whether it is in the patient's best interests to augment the ridge, or whether a more optimal result will be achieved via a prosthesis incorporating a flange.

In the case of single teeth and fixed prostheses it is important to foresee the likely position of the gingival cuff. Previous resorption and certain flap procedures may reposition the papillae further towards the root of the natural tooth. Unless procedures are adopted that will permit the replacement of the papilla, a black triangle will be evident at the adjacent neck of the natural tooth where tissue is absent. This is unsightly when all the other gingival margins appear 'youthful', with typical healthy architecture of the papillae (Fig. 5.9).

An assessment of the depth of the implant head in relation to the mucosal surface in the edentulous span is also important. Where a shouldered abutment is to be used to place the crown margin in the appropriate depth of cuff, it is important to recognize whether the cuff thickness is insufficient to mask the titanium; otherwise, thin mucosa appears black, rather than typically pink. Obviously thin mucosa recognized by palpation or ridge mapping can foreworn the dentist of this risk (Fig. 5.10). Another common difficulty occurs when a template is not used in positioning the implant, or it is found to be impossible to place it in the preferred position. A surgical guide should always be used to position the implant correctly below the intended prosthetic tooth crown. This avoids the problems of masking an abutment that emerges through the mucosa between the planned position of the crowns of the fixed partial restoration.

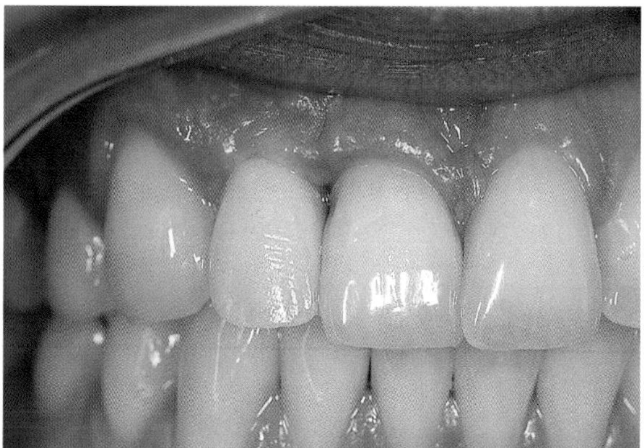

Fig. 5.9 It may prove difficult to restore the gingival architecture around the implant crown, resulting in a deficiency of papilla and a typical small black triangle.

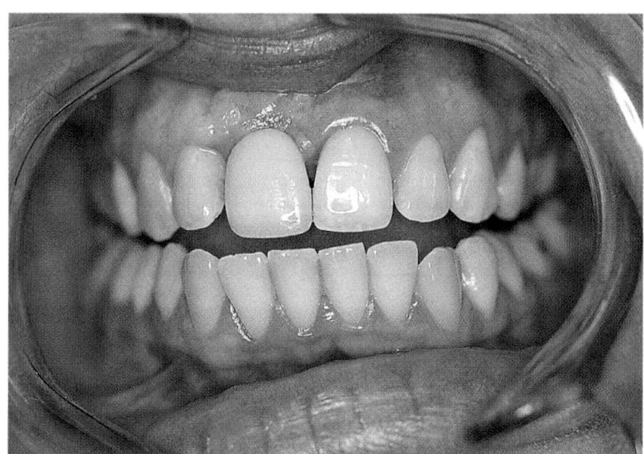

Fig. 5.10 This labial mucosa covering the titanium abutment has a black colour. The presence of a 'high smile-line' would be a disadvantage.

Table 5.7 Avoiding the potential for restorative failure

Factor	Cause
Loss of integration	Placing implants in poor-quality/quantity of bone, using short implants in posterior maxilla Overloading implants. Too few/poor distribution in long span; major discrepancy between arch and implants, creating leverage Parafunction Perimplantitis in partially dentate arch susceptible to bone loss Smoking, previous irradiation
Mechanical problems	Loose screws. Inaccurate fit of components (abutments to implant, abutment to prosthesis). Incorrect linkage (avoid wide platform resisting joint deformation with high loads). Eccentric interferences Loss of cementation. Overloading prosthesis Fracture of components: artificial teeth or extended cantilever in fixed prostheses, retaining clips/caps in removable overdentures
Soft-tissue problems	Cuff hyperplasia/mucosal sinus. Loose abutment screw. Poor oral hygiene. Direct trauma from removable prosthesis

The factors which, singly or in combination, may lead to retorative failure/non-acceptance are listed in Table 5.7.

CONCLUSION

The outcome of several long-term clinical trials with specific dental implants has shown the likelihood of high levels of survival of carefully planned osseointegrated dental implants and prostheses stabilized by them.

As a result, patients are aware that this form of restorative treatment is one they might choose. All dentists must therefore know what information is needed to advise the patient of its appropriateness in their particular case. On occasion this will require a specialist opinion and treatment. However, because of the high cost of treatment and considerations of future maintenance it must be appreciated that the provision of personal or healthcare funding will be important factors in limiting its availability to those who accord it a priority.

REFERENCES

Adell R, Lekholm U, Rockler B, Branemark P-I. A 15-year study of osseointegrated implants in the treatment of the edentulous jaw. Int J Oral Surg 1981; 10: 387–416

Binon PP. Implant and components: entering the new millennium. Int J Oral Maxillofac Implants 2000; 15: 76–94

Brunton PA, Smith PW, McCord JF. Procera all ceramic crowns a new approach to an old problem. Br Dent J 1999; 186: 430–434

Chan MFWY, Narhi TO, de Baat C, Kalk W. Treatment of the atrophic edentulous maxilla with implant-supported overdentures. A review of the literature. Int J Prosthodont 1998; 11: 7–15

Cooper LF, Scurria MS, Lang LA et al. Treatment of edentulism using Astra-Tech implants and ball abutments to retain mandibular overdentures. Int J Oral Maxillofac Implants 1999; 14: 646–653

Davis DM. Implant-stabilized overdentures. Dental Update 1997; 24: 106–109

de Baat C. Success of dental implants in elderly people. A literature review. Gerondontology 2000; 17: 45–48

Denissen HW, Kalk W, van Waas MAJ, van Os JH. Occlusion for maxillary dentures opposing osseointegrated mandibular prostheses. Int J Prosthodont 1993; 6: 446–450

Hobkirk JA, Watson RM. Color atlas and text of dental and maxillo-facial implantology. Barcelona: Mosby-Wolfe, 1995

Jorneus L, Jemt T, Carlsson L. Loads and designs of screw joints for single crowns supported by osseointegrated implants. Int J Oral Maxillofac Implants 1992; 7: 353–359

Lang BR, Razzoog ME. Lingualised integration: Tooth molds and an occlusal scheme for edentulous implant patients. Implant Dent 1992; 1: 204–211

Lekholm U, Gunne J, Henry P et al. Survival of the Branemark implant in partially edentulous jaws. A 10-year prospective multicenter study. Int J Oral Maxillofac Implants 1999; 14: 639–645

Priest G. Single tooth implants and their role in preserving remaining teeth. A 10-year survival study. Int J Oral Maxillofac Implants 1999; 14: 181–188

Triplett RG, Schow SR, Laskin DM. Oral and maxillofacial surgery advances in implant dentistry. Int J Oral Maxillofac Implants 2000; 15: 47–55

Watson RM, Davis DM. Follow up and maintenance of implant supported prostheses: a comparison of 20 complete mandibular overdentures and 20 complete mandibular fixed cantilever prostheses. Br Dent J 1996; 181: 321–327

Appendix
Case planning exercises

Included in this Appendix are 14 cases. Outline scenarios are presented with a list of potential treatment options. The scenarios are followed by comments on these options and an explanation of the treatment(s) carried out.

A broad range has been included, including one patient who is edentulous but for whom the options might include implant-supported bridgework.

We do not expect all readers to agree with the treatment carried out, but we feel that the scenarios offer good learning opportunities.

GWENT HEALTHCARE NHS TRUST
LIBRARY
ROYAL GWENT HOSPITAL
NEWPORT

Planning Case 1

Mr B. H. – Age 54 years	
Occupation	Engineer
Complaint	Not able to eat with comfort and appearance was an embarrassment.
Past medical history	Reflux oesophagitis (R_x lansoprazole 20 mg). History of surgery for masseteric hypertrophy – still suffers from trismus (10 mm opening anteriorly).
Past dental history	Reasonable dental attender. Had several sets of P/– dentures made over the years; his lower two-part denture has lost one section and no denture has been worn for 3 years.
Findings	OH good and caries present in 47. No BPE>1. Marked loss in facial height noticed (Fig. C1.1). Good bone levels (see DPT – Fig. C1.2). Figures C1.3 and C1.4 show upper and lower arches at presentation and upper acrylic tissue-borne RPD. Fractured MO restoration 47 with chipped buccal cusps.

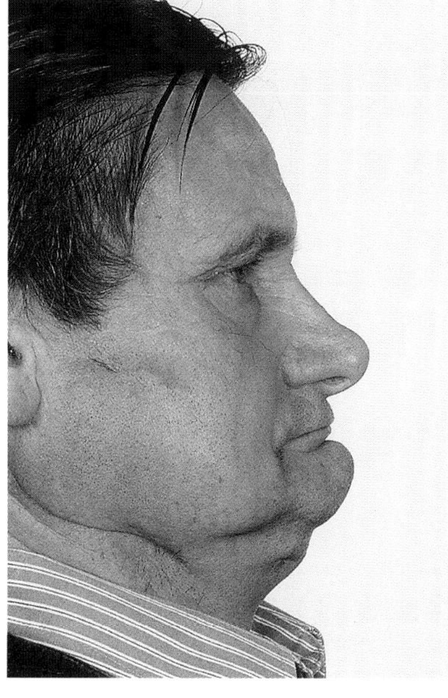

Fig. C1.1

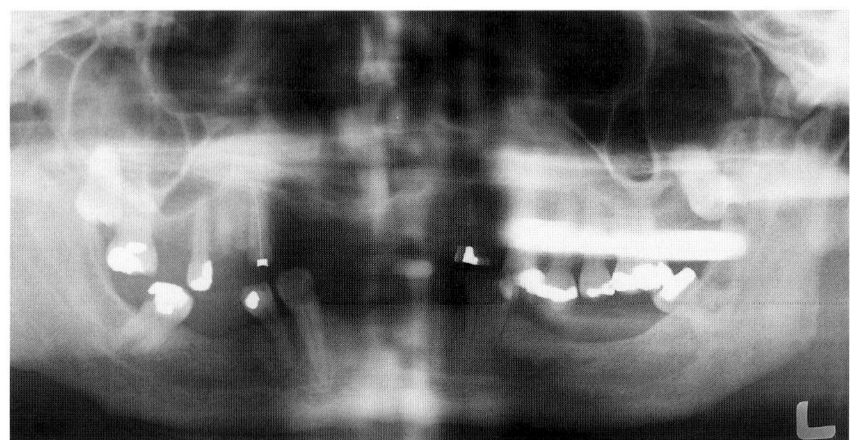

Fig. C1.2

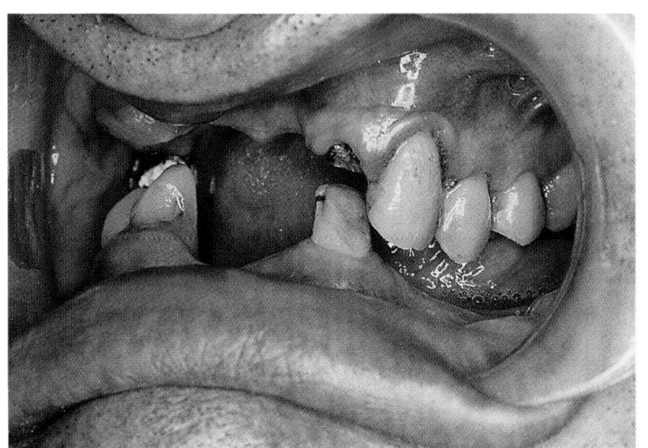

Fig. C1.3

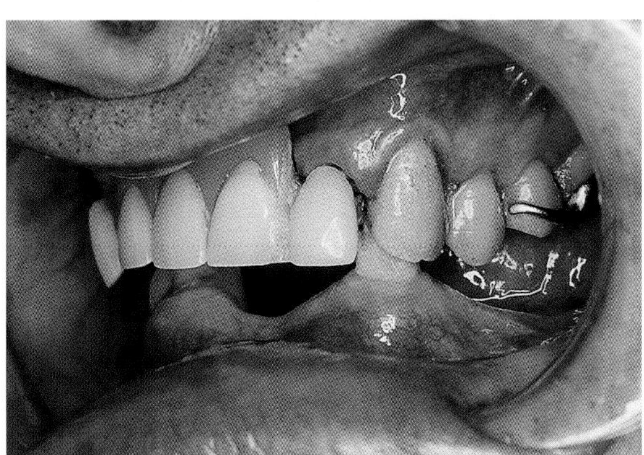

Fig. C1.4

Charting

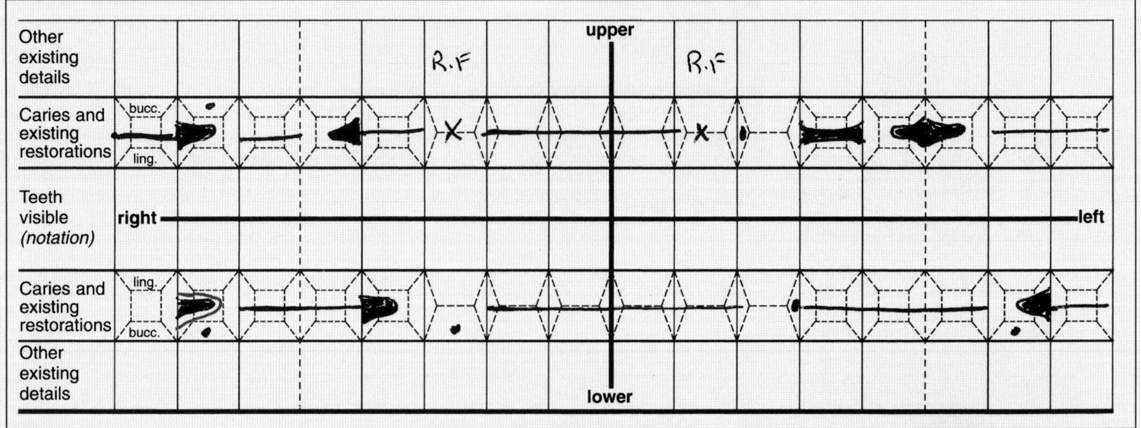

Chart 1.1

Social history Non-smoker, non-drinker, likes hill walking.

TREATMENT OPTIONS

1. Do nothing
2. Make replacement P/P
3. Make P/- and fixed mandibular prosthesis
4. Implant-retained prostheses
5. Render edentulous and give C/- and -/C.

Comments

1. Do nothing: not a realistic option – patient is keen to retain teeth and 13 and 22 are sound overdenture abutments
2. Make replacement P/P: problems of major connector selection for –/P, and interocclusal space is at a premium (Fig. C1.5).
3. Make P/– and fixed mandibular prosthesis (selected option – see below)
4. Implant-retained prostheses might be considered but space is very limited owing to trismus.
5. Render edentulous/decoronate teeth and give C/C (either conventional or over-denture). Patient did not wish to even consider this!

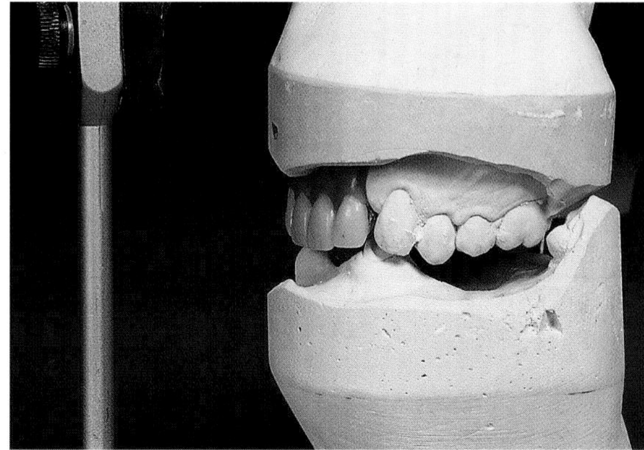

Fig. C1.5

TREATMENT AGREED

1. Gold shell crown 47.
2. Maxillary RPD – outline drawing for planning is shown in Fig. C1.6. The inserted denture is shown in Fig. C1.7 (N.B. gold shell crown 47 has not yet been prepared/inserted).

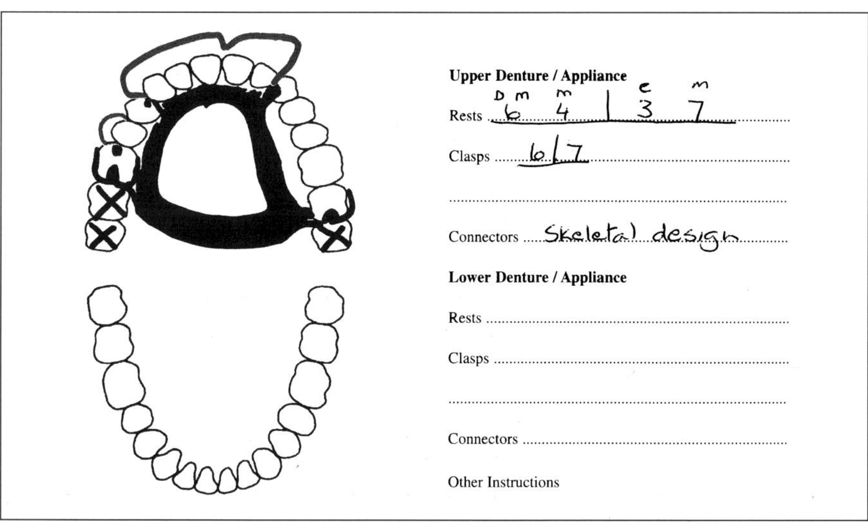

Upper Denture / Appliance

Rests D 6 m, m 4 | c 3, m 7

Clasps 6 | 7

Connectors Skeletal design

Lower Denture / Appliance

Rests

Clasps

Connectors

Other Instructions

Fig. C1.6

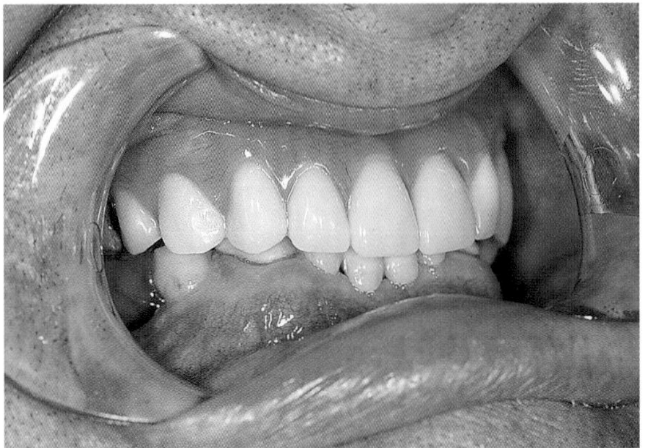

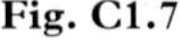
Fig. C1.7

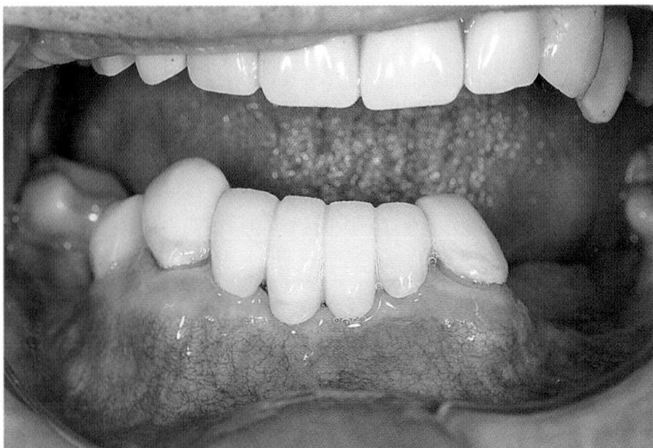

Fig. C1.8

3. Resin-bonded ceramic bridge 43-33, with a labial path of insertion.
4. In effect this was a labial veneer bridge (now in place 2.8 years) (Fig. C1.8).
5. The difference in the appearance and in patient confidence was striking (Fig. C1.9).

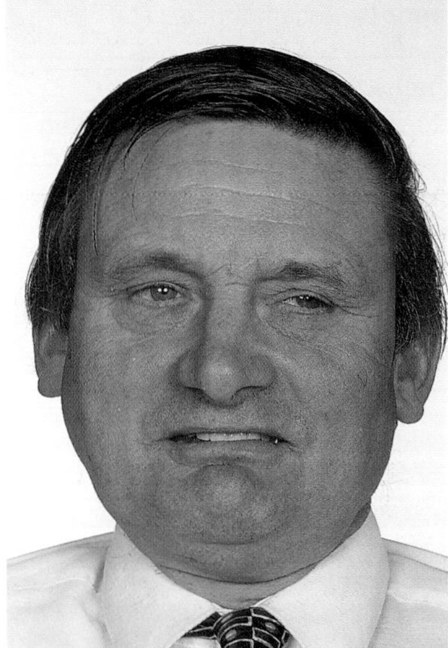

Fig. C1.9

Planning Case 2

Mr E. C. – Age 64 years	
Occupation	Retired newsagent
Complaint	No longer able to bite satisfactorily: 'lost my bite'.
Past medical history	Type II diabetes (tablet controlled R_x 20 mg) Prescribed antihypertensive and analgesics for general aches.
Past dental history	Reasonable dental attender. Had one mandibular RPD made 2 years previously but was not happy with appearance or function.
Findings	BPE 1 in all sextants except 2 in lower left sextant. Marked Class III appearance (Fig. C2.1). Good bone levels except 34/5 region (see DPT – Fig. C2.2). Figures C2.3 (mirror view) and C2.4 show upper and lower arches at presentation. Metal ceramic crowns (MCC) provided 12, 11, 21 and 22 18 months previously. OH fair and one leaking restoration, namely 12 (distal). 'Biting still a problem!'
Social history	Keen golfer, but had to buy three pairs of (increasingly larger) golf shoes over a 2-year period. Likes 'occasional cigar and a beer'.

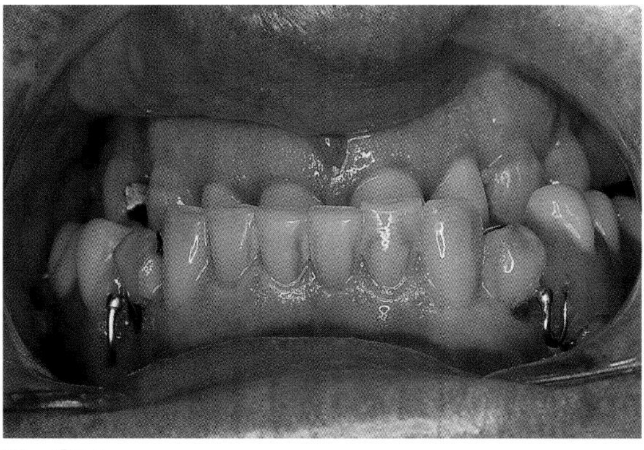

Fig. C2.1

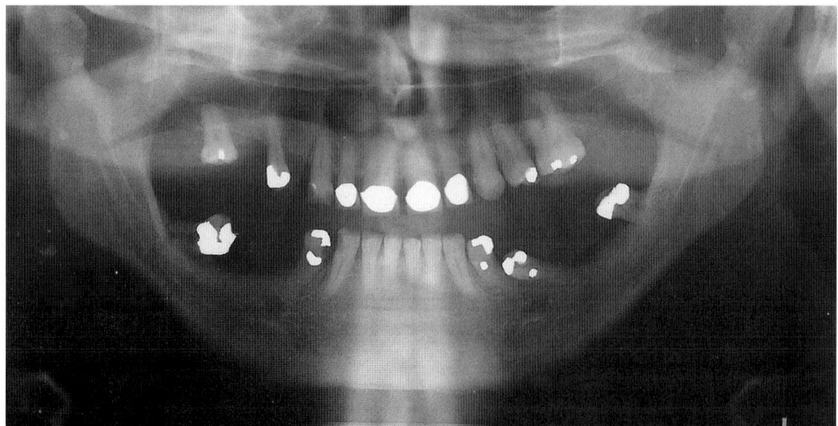

Fig. C2.2

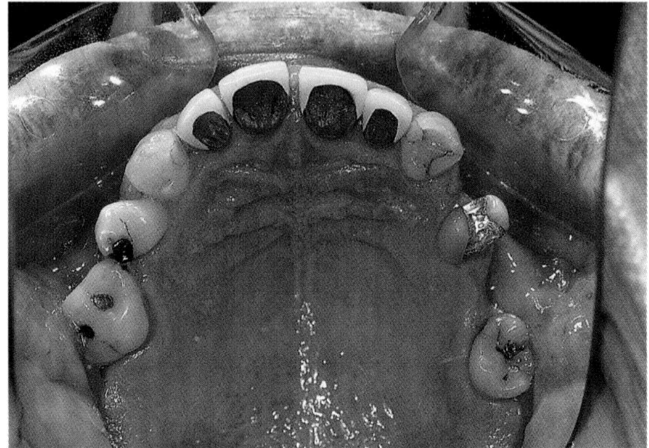

Fig. C2.3 Mirror view.

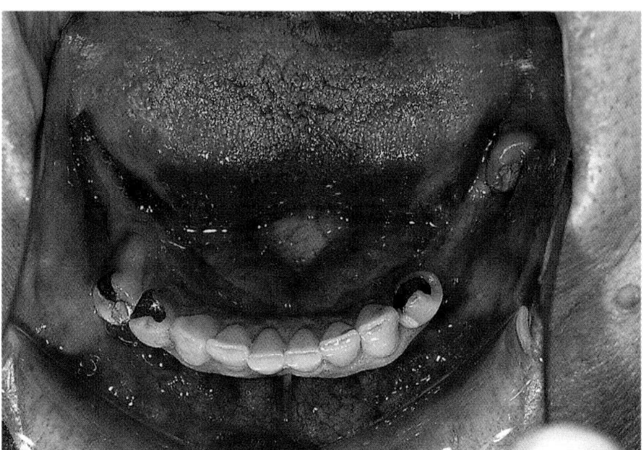

Fig. C2.4

Charting

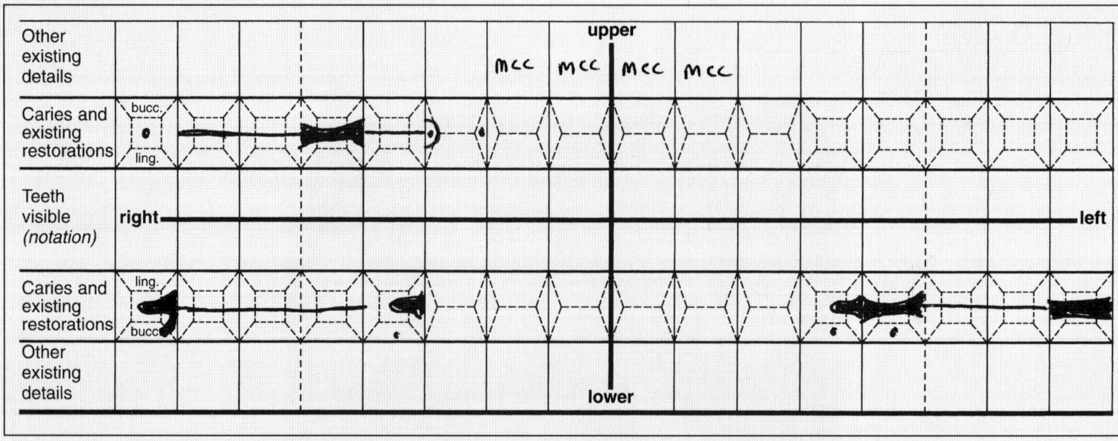

								upper								
Other existing details							mcc	mcc	mcc	mcc						
Caries and existing restorations (bucc. / ling.)																
Teeth visible *(notation)*	right															left
Caries and existing restorations (ling. / bucc.)																
Other existing details									lower							

Chart 2.1

TREATMENT OPTIONS

1. Do nothing other than primary therapy (restore 12 and oral hygiene and oral hygiene instruction (OH/OHI)).
2. Make mandibular RPD plus primary therapy.
3. Make a fixed mandibular prosthesis plus primary therapy.
4. Implant-retained prostheses plus primary therapy.
5. Orthodontic treatment to give edge-to-edge occlusion after primary therapy.
6. Refer to consultant in oral medicine and reappraise assessment of pituitary function – plus primary therapy.

TREATMENT CARRIED OUT

1. Basic OH and RPD.
2. Provide a mandibular RPD. Outline drawing for planning is shown in Fig. C2.6 and fitted RPD in Fig. C2.7.
3. Return to dentist for continuing care.

Comments

1. Do nothing: will not address the patient's problem. Even if no dentistry is carried out, the fact that the patient is emphatic he had no anterior crossbite before suggests that medical investigations are required.
2. This may be all that is required, after results of pituitary assay etc. are known.
3. May restore a few missing teeth but the inclination of the remaining teeth, the bone levels around 34 and the need to alter the mandibular plane (Fig. C2.5) raise doubts over this.
4. May be a consideration but the patient wished no oral surgery.
5. Even if feasible, the patient refused to contemplate fixed therapy or any form of oral and maxillofacial surgery.
6. This was done. The patient was diagnosed as suffering from acromegaly. He underwent surgery on the pituitary gland and his diabetes, generalized aches and hypertension resolved.

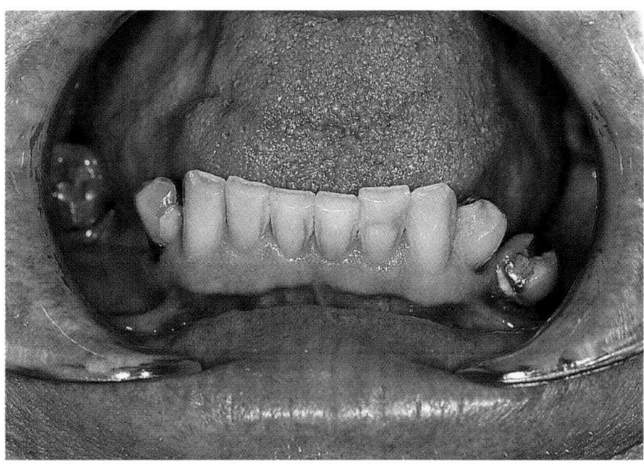

Fig. C2.5

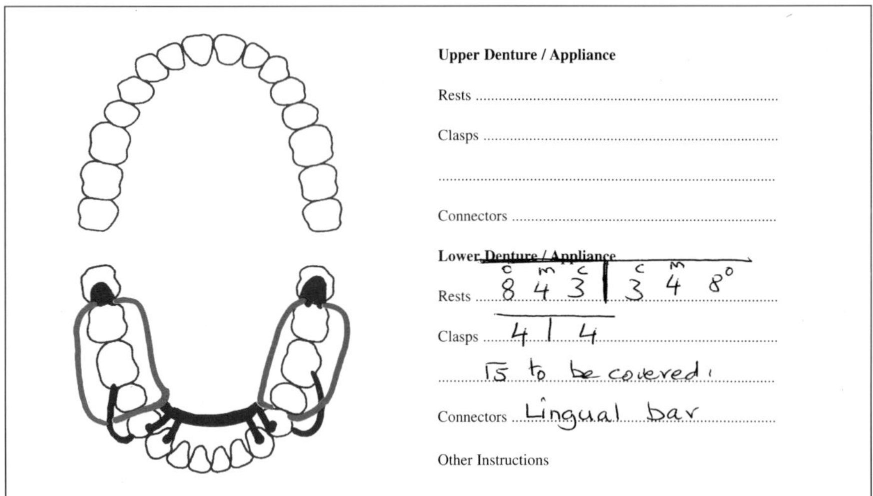

Upper Denture / Appliance

Rests ....

Clasps ....

....

Connectors ....

Lower Denture / Appliance

Rests 8 4 3 | 3 4 8

Clasps 4 | 4

5 to be covered

Connectors Lingual bar

Other Instructions

Fig. C2.6

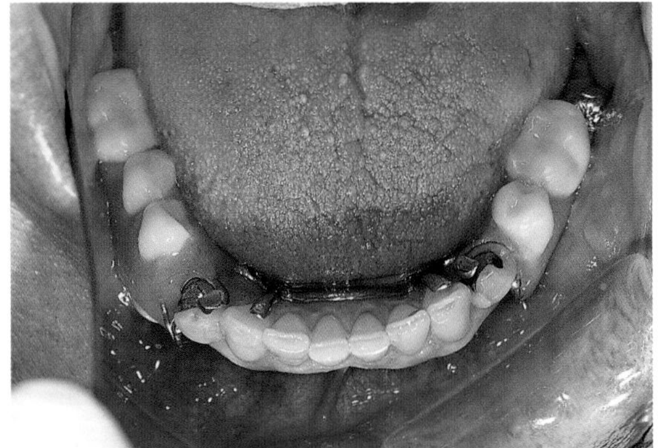

Fig. C2.7

Planning Case 3

Mrs M. P. – Age 48 years	
Occupation	Teacher
Complaint	Not able to eat with comfort and wishes to replace lost teeth for appearance's sake.
Past medical history	Hayfever.
Past dental history	Had two remaining maxillary molars removed 1 year ago. Since then, has not been able to wear her partial denture. Reasonable regular dental attender; wears mandibular RPD (Fig. C3.1).
Findings	OH not exemplary, BPE 1 in all relevant sextants. No intermaxillary space between 37 and 47 and the opposing ridge (Fig. C3.2).

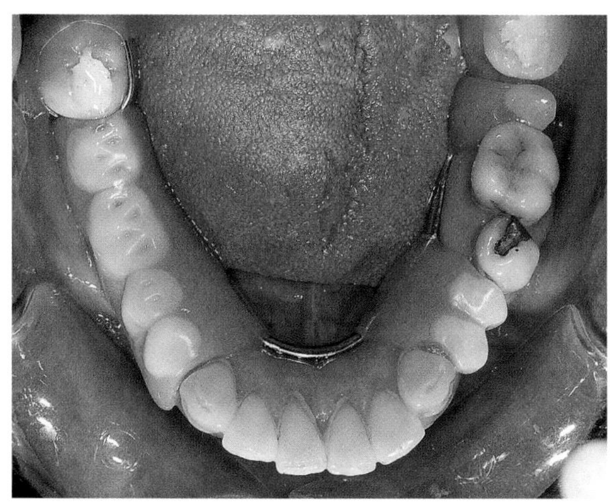

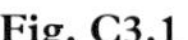
Fig. C3.1

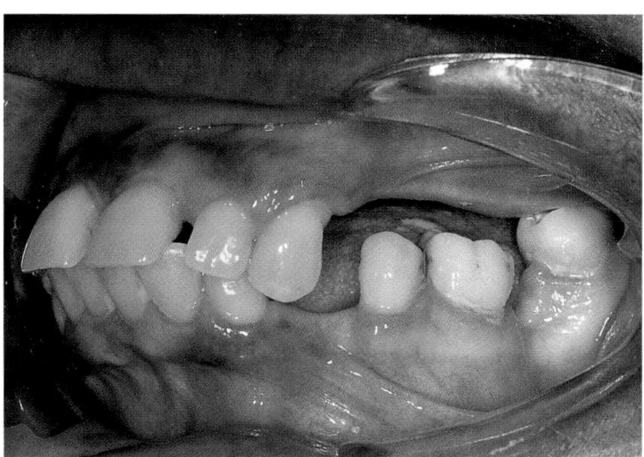
Fig. C3.2

Charting

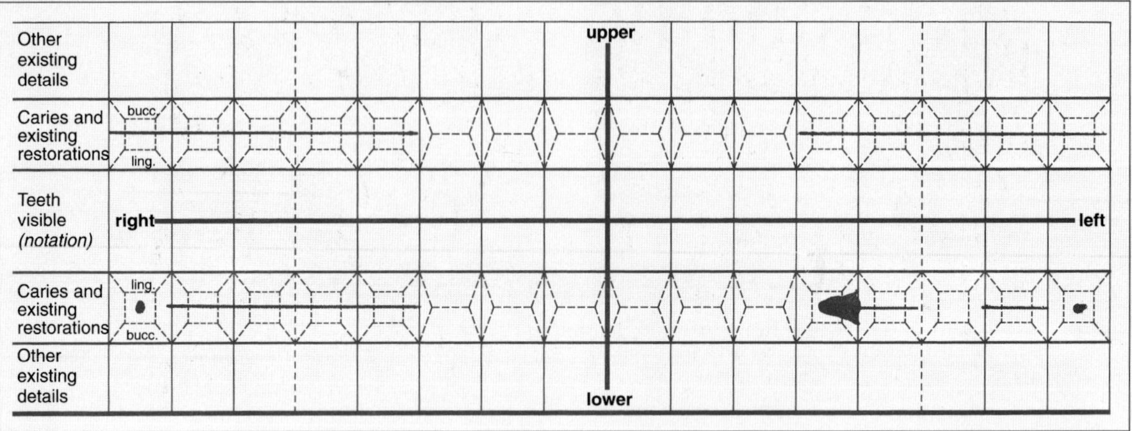

Chart 3.1

Social history	Smoked 30 per day. Does not wish any major surgery, as she objects to blood transfusions.

TREATMENT OPTIONS

1. Do nothing other than OH/OHI
2. Make replacement removable prostheses at present OVD after OH/OHI
3. Make replacement removable prostheses at increased OVD after OH/OHI
4. Insert implants and provide fixed/ removable prostheses after OH/OHI
5. Remove remaining teeth and provide C/C.

Comments

1. Do nothing not an option: the patient is concerned over function and appearance.
2. Removable prostheses at present OVD: a real option, but all four canine teeth have no appreciable undercuts available for retention. OH/OHI is required.
3. Removable prostheses at increased OVD: also an option, same comments valid.
4. Implant therapy: would involve surgery to raise the floor of the maxillary antrum (Fig. C3.3). Patient smokes and does not wish to consider surgery.
5. Render edentulous: not a sensible suggestion.

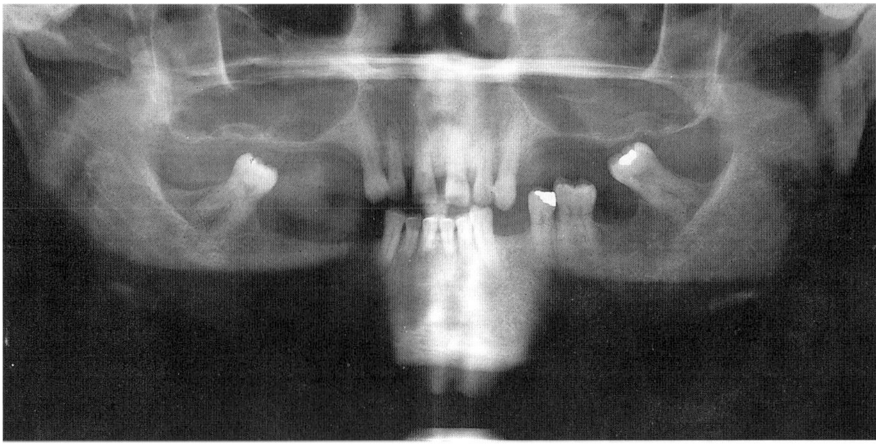

Fig. C3.3

TREATMENT PROVIDED

1. OH and OHI plus monitoring and counselling over smoking.
2. Upper splint to raise OVD to determine whether patient could tolerate an increase in OVD – she could not.
3. To provide space for the maxillary denture, elective endodontics was carried out on 27 and 47 and the crowns reduced in height. Composite additions (0.25 mm undercuts) were made to the distolabial surfaces of 33 and 43 to provide retention for direct retainers (Fig. C3.4).
4. To provide good retention and stability for the maxillary RPD, 13 and 23 were prepared for metal-ceramic crowns with guide surfaces on the distal aspects plus Ceka extracoronal attachments. The crowns were milled to have a mesial rest and a palatal channel to house the indirect retainer and its minor connector. A U-shaped maxillary RPD was made (see Fig. C3.5 for outline planning drawings) with a posterior palatal strap (meshwork placed to enable relining when required) and a planned path of insertion to augment indirect retainers (Figs C3.6 and C3.7).

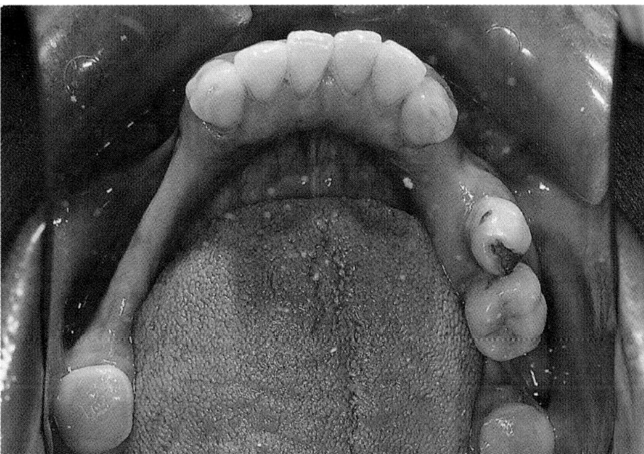

Fig. C3.4 Mirror view.

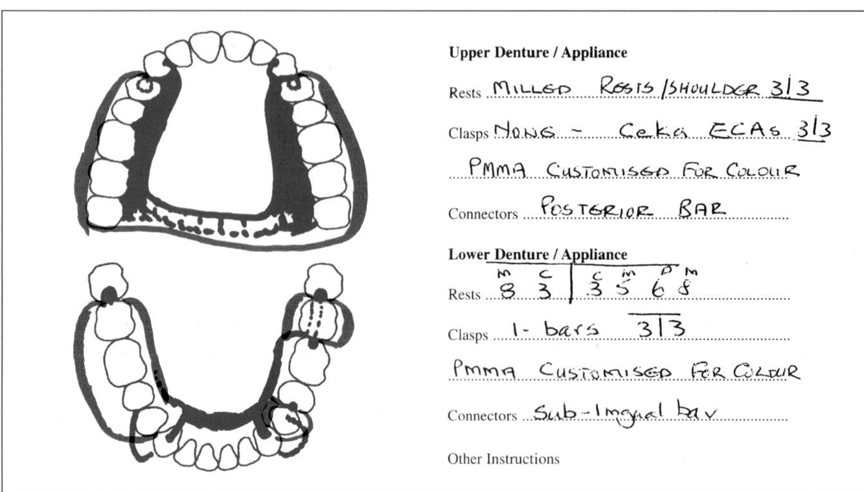

Upper Denture / Appliance

Rests MILLED RESTS /SHOULDER 3|3

Clasps NONE - Ceka ECAs 3|3

PMMA CUSTOMISED FOR COLOUR

Connectors POSTERIOR BAR

Lower Denture / Appliance

Rests M C | C M P M — 8 3 | 3 5 6 8

Clasps I- bars 3|3

PMMA CUSTOMISED FOR COLOUR

Connectors Sub-lingual bar

Other Instructions

Fig. C3.5

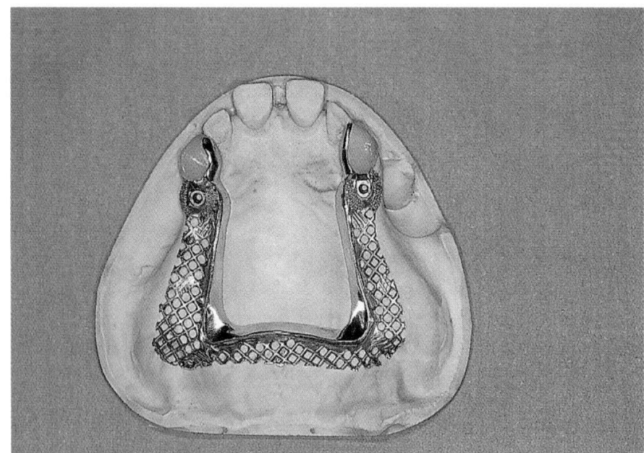

Fig. C3.6

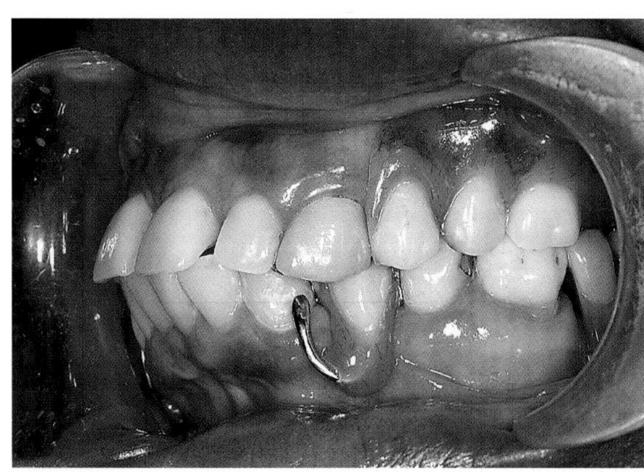

Fig. C3.7

Planning Case 4

Mrs J. W. – Age 25 years	
Occupation	Housewife
Complaint	Unsightly denture.
Past medical history	Sickle cell trait.
Past dental history	Regular attender. Moderately high DMF score. Lost 21 and 22 as a result of a car crash 3 years ago. Was given an immediate insertion (I.I.) RPD which she now wears – it is a mucosa-borne RPD (Fig. C4.1).
Findings	OH fair and BPE of 1 in the three maxillary sextants and nil in the mandibular sextants. There is a carious cavity present in the distal of 12. (Fig. C4.2).

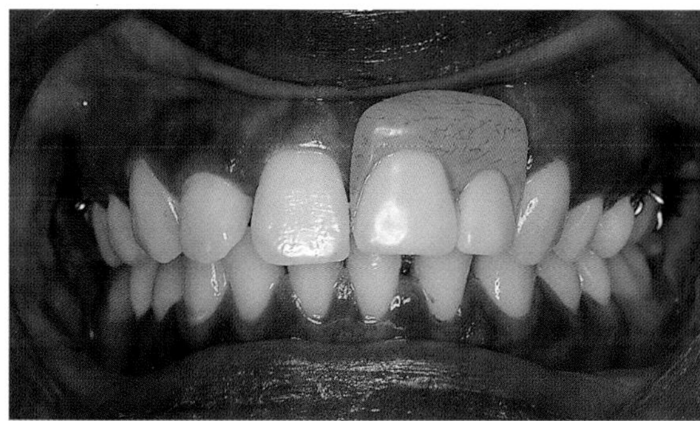

Fig. C4.1

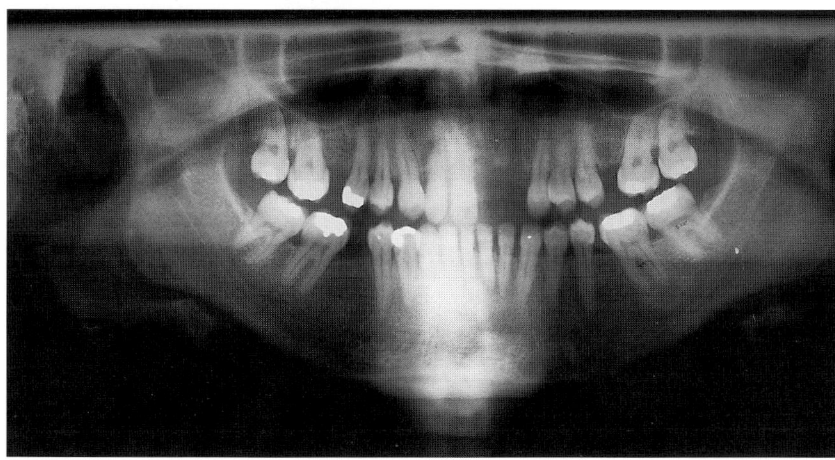

Fig. C4.2

Charting

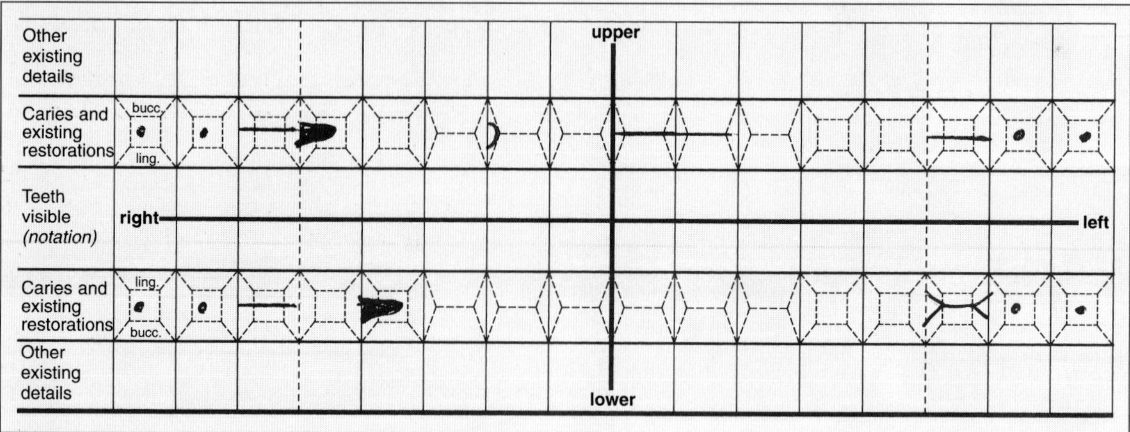

Chart 4.1

Social history Teacher, non-smoker and has now 'abandoned eating chocolate'.

TREATMENT OPTIONS

1. Do nothing (other than OH/OHI)
2. Replace RPD plus primary (simple conservative and periodontal) therapy
3. Restore with fixed prosthesis plus other primary therapy
4. Restore missing teeth with implant-borne prosthesis(es) after primary therapy
5. Rendering edentulous is not a sensible option here.

Comments

1. Do nothing: not a professional option. The RPD has long since served its purpose. Small cavity 12 requires attention (Fig. C4.3).
2. Removable option plus primary therapy: a real option.
3. Fixed option. Problematic using conventional means owing to spacing in this Afro-Caribbean young woman (with the exception of 12, the remaining anterior teeth are unrestored.
4. Implants: might be feasible if ridges were of sufficient dimension. However, the labiopalatal width of the ridge in the edentulous area was only 2.5 mm. As general anaesthesia would in all probability be required, the implant option was not pursued.

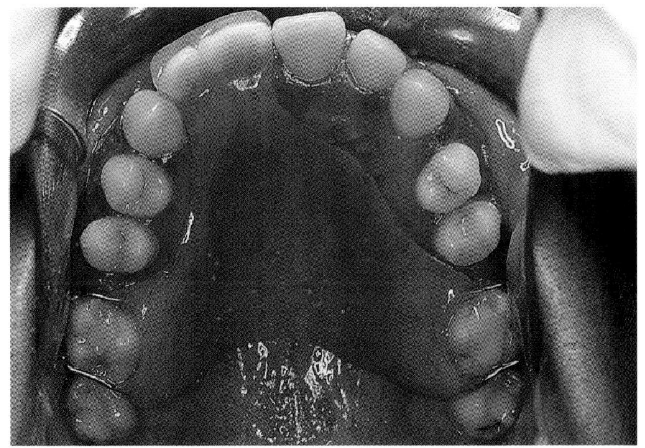

Fig. C4.3 Mirror view.

TREATMENT PROVIDED

1. OH, OHI and monitoring.
2. 12 (distal) composite restoration.
3. Cobalt-chromium based RPD provided – see Fig. C4.4 for outline drawing for planning. For reasons of appearance plus retention, it was decided to use a planned path of insertion to enable good restoration of the interdental papilla (Fig. C4.5).

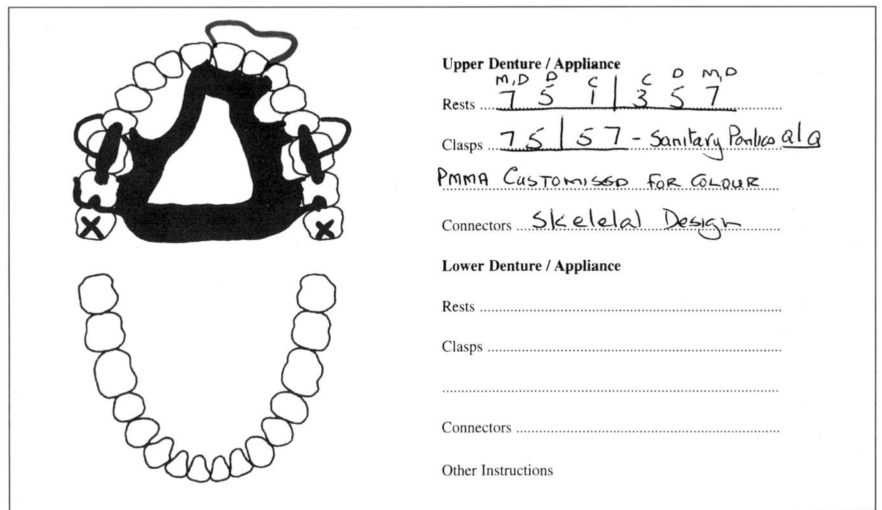

Upper Denture / Appliance

Rests: M,D 7, D 5, C 1 | C 3, D 5, M,D 7

Clasps: 7 5 | 5 7 - Sanitary Pontics a|a

PMMA CUSTOMISED FOR COLOUR

Connectors: Skelelal Design

Lower Denture / Appliance

Rests ....

Clasps ....

....

Connectors ....

Other Instructions

Fig. C4.4

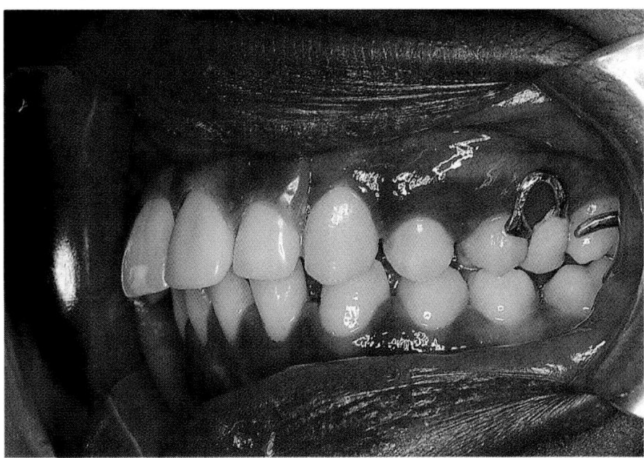

Fig. C4.5

Planning Case 5

Mrs M.R. – Age 52 years	
Occupation	Lawyer
Complaint	Mobile and painful upper right lateral incisor.
Past medical history	Slight angina and is prescribed Mogadon 'as a sleeping tablet'.
Past dental history	Had a fixed prosthesis to replace 15 and 14 2 years previously. Post crown on 12.
Findings	No BPE>1. 12 had been apicectomied 2 years previously. Residual infection apparent and secondary caries present on root. Sinus present on labial aspect of root. Poor fit of crown (Fig. C5.1). OH fair, bridge margins acceptable on abutments (A) 17 and 13. Fig. C5.1

Charting

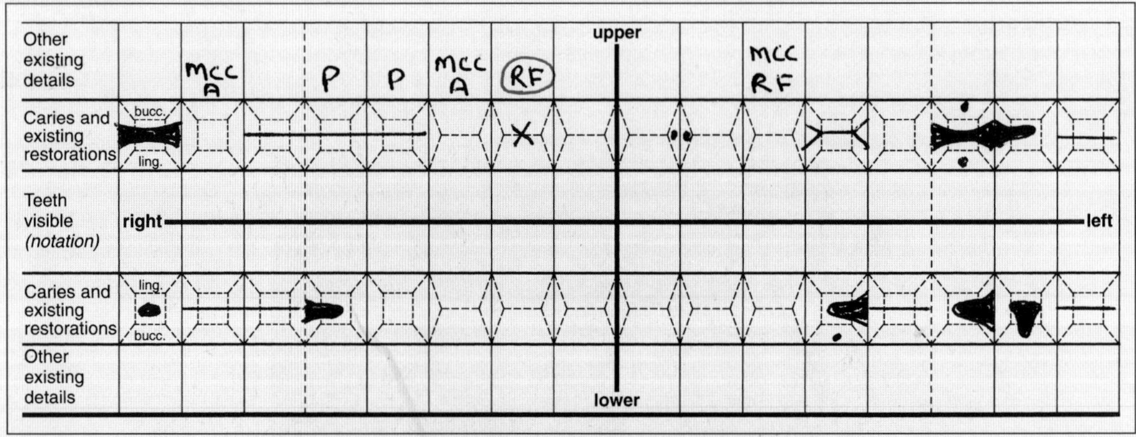

Chart 5.1

Social history	Non-smoker, well informed about dental care. Has a history of being a severe retcher when wearing maxillary RPD, hence fixed prosthesis.

TREATMENT OPTIONS

1. Do nothing
2. Replace post crown
3. Extract post crown and provide immediate insertion (I.I.) RPD and then provide a definitive RPD
4. Extract post crown, provide I.I. RPD and then make a fixed prosthesis to restore lost lateral incisor
5. Extract post crown and provide I.I. RPD, and then provide an implant-supported prosthesis (crown)
6. Rendering edentulous is neither a realistic nor a sensible option!

Comments

1. Do nothing. Given the presence of pain, mobility and the sinus associated with 12, this is not an option.
2. Replace post crown 12. This is not sensible, owing to the amount of periapical infection, the caries present on the root face and the unfavourable crown:root ratio.
3. Extract 12 and an II RPD is a social necessity. However, this patient does not wish to have a definitive prosthesis, owing to previous retching problem.
4. Extract 12, provide II RPD and then provide a fixed option. The fixed bridge 16-13 is perfectly acceptable and 11 is unrestored (Fig. C5.2). This means that either pristine teeth are sacrificed or a good bridge is destroyed and a new and larger bridge is provided.
5. Extract post crown and provide I.I. RPD and then provide an implant-supported prosthesis (crown). This is a real option following healing of the extraction site.

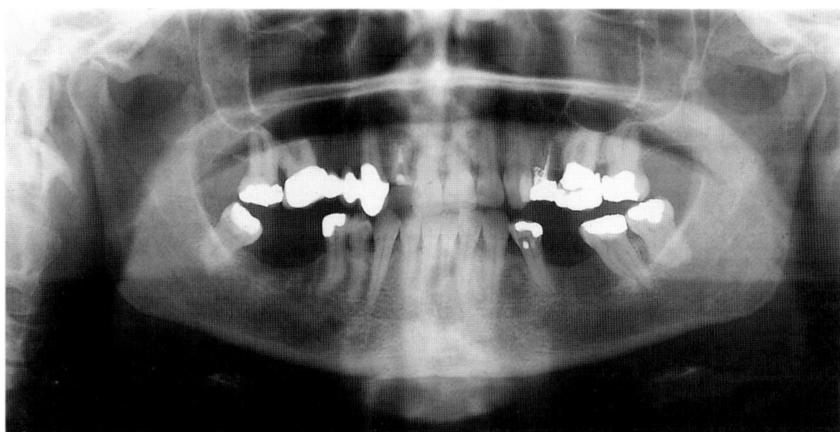

Fig. C5.2

TREATMENT PROVIDED

1. 12 was extracted and an II RPD provided in the form of a Manchester veneer. Composite additions were made to 13 (mesial) and 11 (distal), and a labial veneer with a replacing 12 provided (Figs. C5.3 and C5.4).
2. A Frialit 2 implant was subsequently placed and a Procera crown placed 6 months later to complete the restoration (Figs. C5.5 and C5.6).

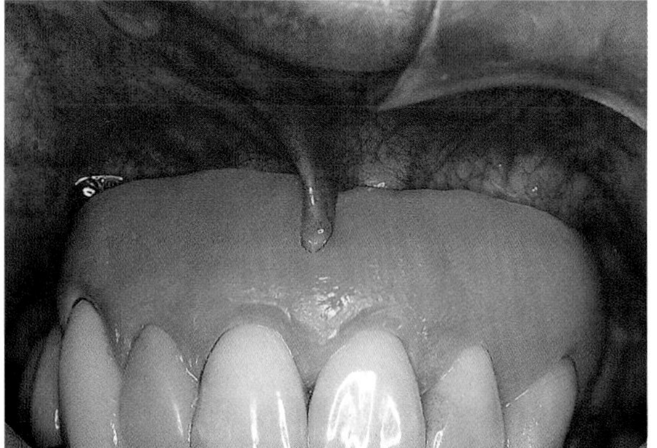

Fig. C5.3

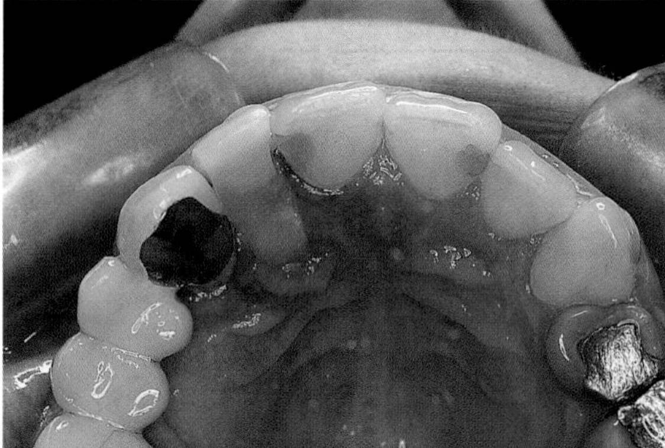

Fig. C5.4

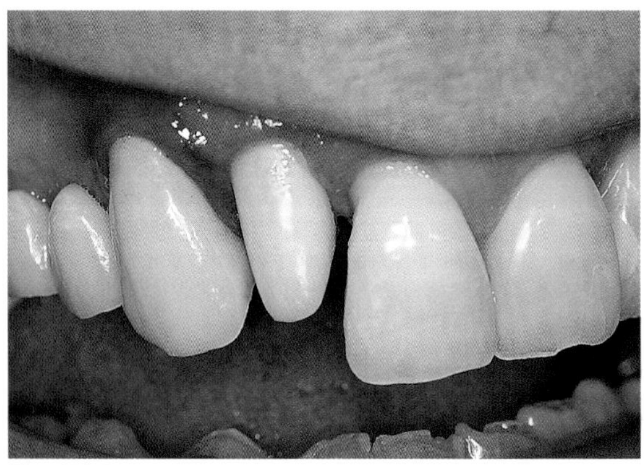

Fig. C5.5

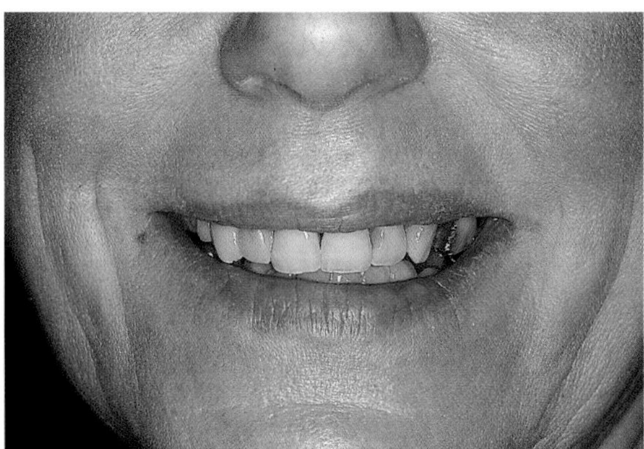

Fig. C5.6

Planning Case 6

Miss H.T. – Age 20 years	
Occupation	University student
Complaint	Appearance owing to missing lateral incisor.
Past medical history	Asthma as a child, eczema.
Past dental history	Referred by GDP re suitability for dental implant to replace RPD following previous orthodontic treatment for missing lateral incisor (Fig. C6.1).
Findings	Excellent dentition with good plaque control. BPE of 0 in all sextants. 22 is a small tooth. Right lateral space small with some alveolar concavity. Normal overbite. Arch only displayed in smiling. Diastema distal to 13.

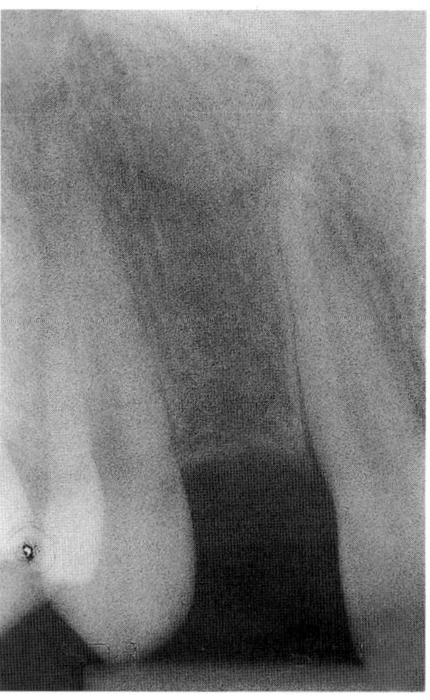

Fig. C6.1

Charting

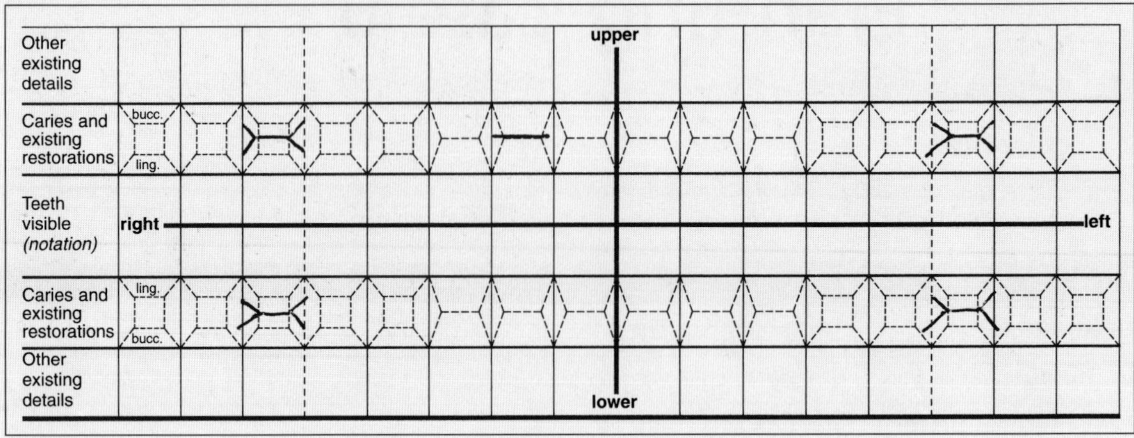

Chart 6.1

Social history Non-smoker, intelligent patient, keen to have an aesthetic result.

TREATMENT OPTIONS

1. Orthodontics to close space and accept restored occlusion
2. Orthodontics to align and create a space of 4–5 mm and restore this with an RPD
3. Orthodontics to align and create a space of 4–5 mm and restore this with a fixed option (could be a conventional fixed–fixed or cantilever design, or a resin-bonded bridge)
4. Conventional cantilever bridge
(Rendering edentulous is clearly not an option here.)

Comments

1. Doing nothing is not an option here.
2. Patient motivation against deterioration of the status quo is high.
3. Orthodontics to close space. As the maxillary centre line is likely to shift this would result in an asymmetric arch, the appearance of which would be unacceptable to the patient.
4. Even after orthodontic space creation the placement of an RPD is likely to place abutment teeth and underlying mucosa at risk in the long term.
5. A conventional bridge would be severely destructive of intact teeth, a resin-bonded bridge would disturb the patient's occlusion and would also have a detrimental effect on the colour.
6. The implant is the most natural option, as it replaces one lost dental element and sustains the bone volume.

TREATMENT CARRIED OUT – AFTER ADDITIONAL ORTHODONTICS

1. Surgical stage 1: an 18 mm, 3.75 mm Branemark implant was placed using a prepared template. The small labial dehiscence was covered with Bio-oss and Bioguide membrane. Tooth-borne transitional RPD inserted.
2. Surgical stage 2: 6 months later a flap was raised to enhance the gingival position of the 5 mm healing abutment (Fig. C6.2).
3. Transitional RPD fractured and was repaired.
4. Cera-one abutment 1 mm collar (Fig. C6.3) and ceramic crown provided (Figs. C6.4, and C6.5).

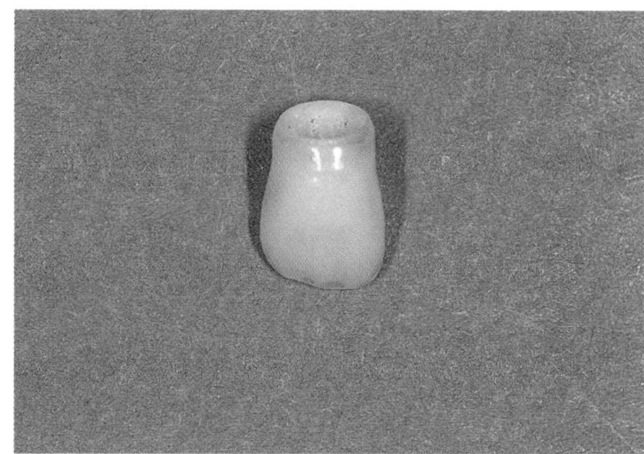

Fig. C6.4

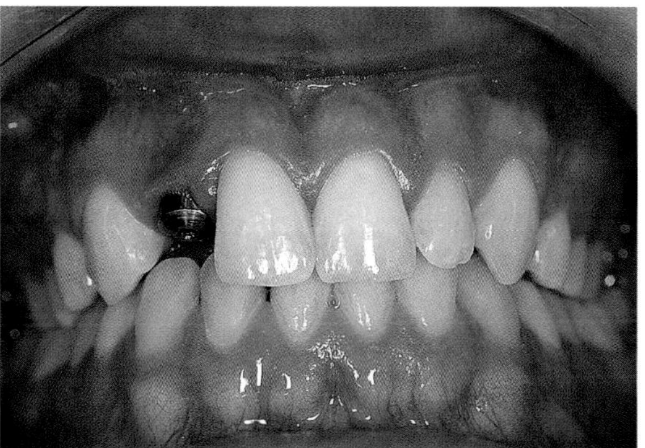

Fig. C6.2

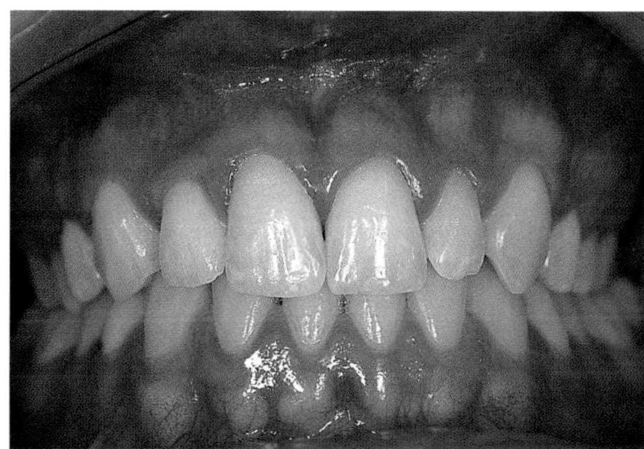

Fig. C6.5

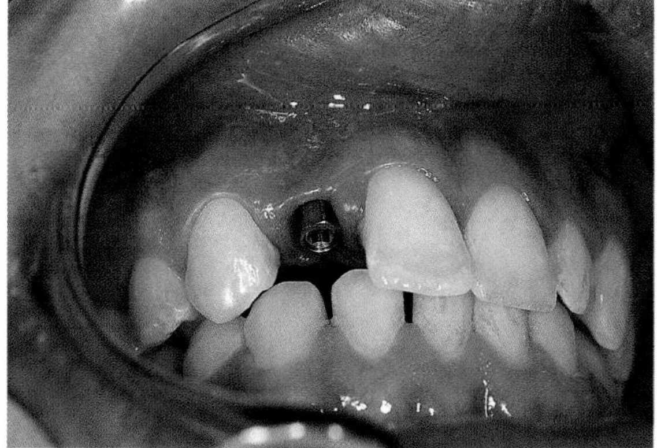

Fig. C6.3

Planning Case 7

Miss J.H. – Age 30 years	
Occupation	Nurse
Complaint	Unstable and unsightly appearance of RPD. Traumatic tooth loss (upper left incisor canine and premolars – road traffic accident).
Past medical history	Nil relevant.
Past dental history	Regular dental attender. RTA 8 months previously resulted in a Le Fort I maxillary fracture and loss 21, 22, 23, 24 and 25. Immediate RPD provided and patient is wearing an acrylic RPD which is 5 months old and very unstable (Fig. C7.1).
Findings	Excellent dentition, well intercuspated and no severe overbite (Fig. C7.2). Marginal gingivitis associated with RPD palatally. Very good plaque control, with no BPE>1. Residual ridge resorption has resulted in a long span with good alveolar form (see Fig. C7.2). Adequate vertical space between ridge and opposing teeth. Radiographs indicate good bone volume.

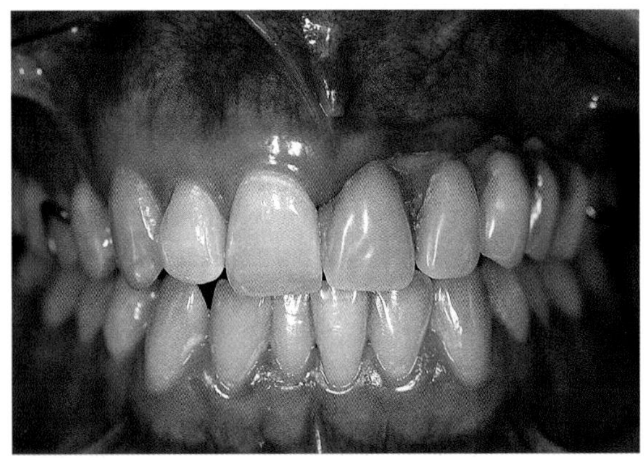

Fig. C7.1

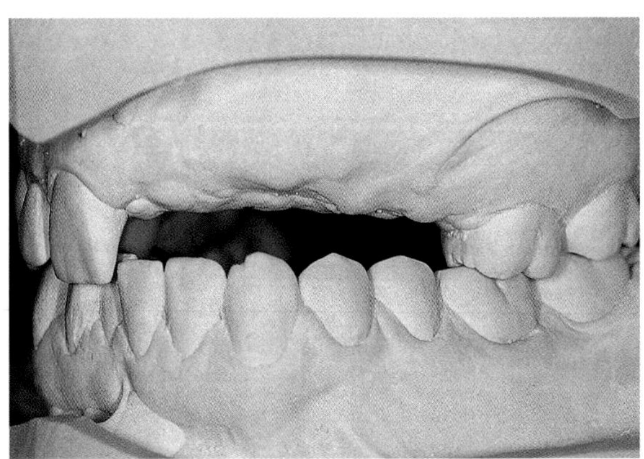

Fig. C7.2

Charting

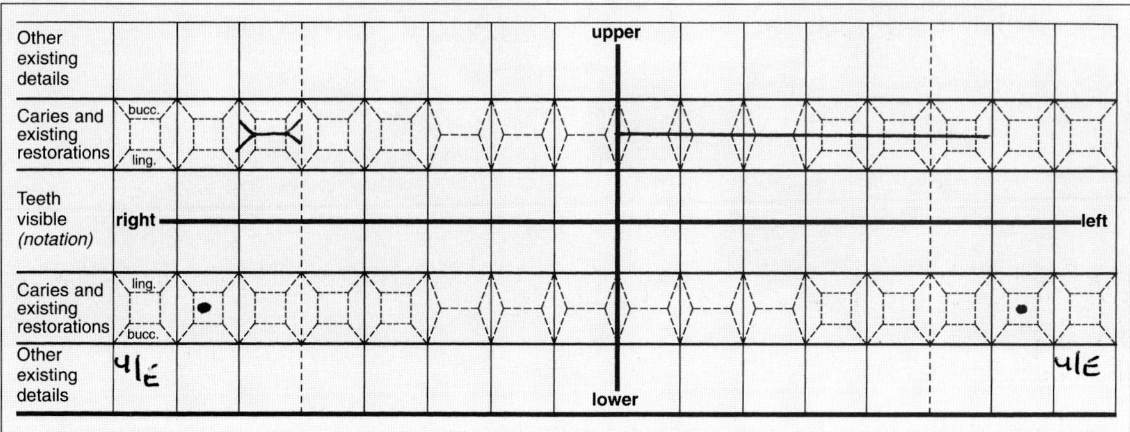

Chart 7.1

Social history Non-smoker, very health conscious.

TREATMENT OPTIONS

1. Doing nothing is not really an option here (see below)
2. RPD – metal frame, replacing transitional acrylic denture
3. Fixed partial implant prostheses with four 13 or 10 mm standard diameter implants (Rendering edentulous cannot be seen as an option here.)

Comments

1. Delaying treatment might result in overeruption of opposing teeth, even if an RPD is worn.
2. Problems common to all RPDs, e.g. clasps and saddle junction are unaesthetic.
3. Continued alveolar remodelling makes rebasing of cobalt-chromium frame more problematic (see Planning Case 3 (MP)).
4. Long span creates problems of retention for a removable and fixed option. For fixed options the remaining teeth are intact and a conventional bridge would be destructive to sound tooth tissue.
5. There is a high probability of failure from occlusal forces for the fixed and removable options.

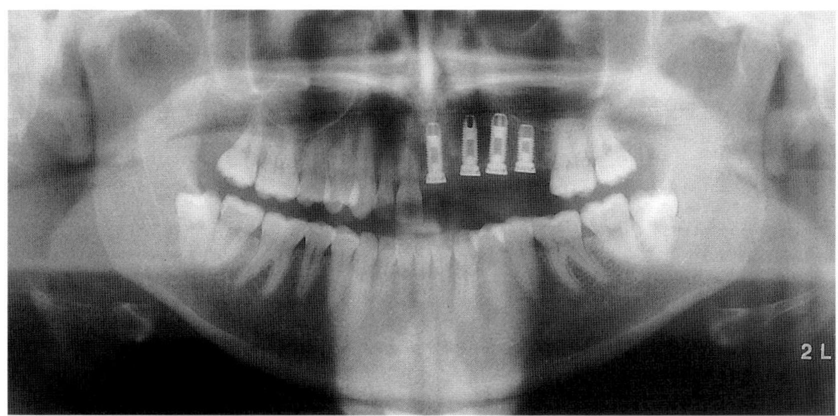

Fig. C7.3

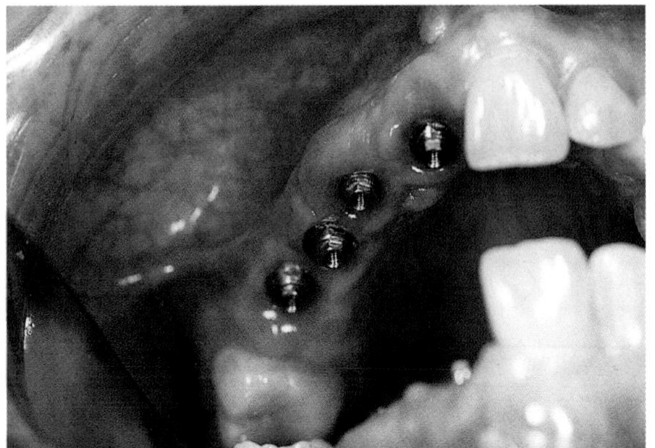
Fig. C7.4 Mirror view from above.

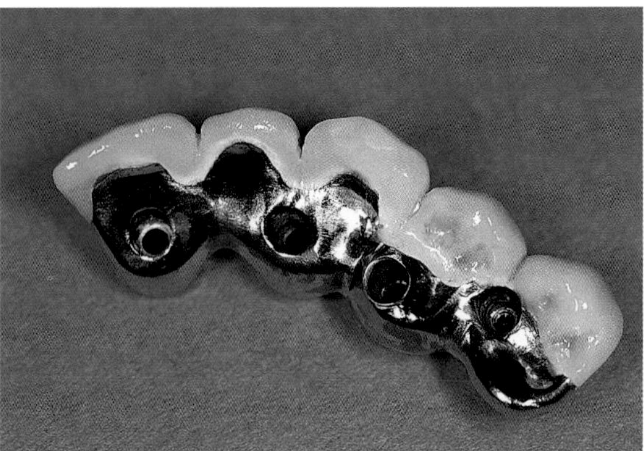
Fig. C7.5

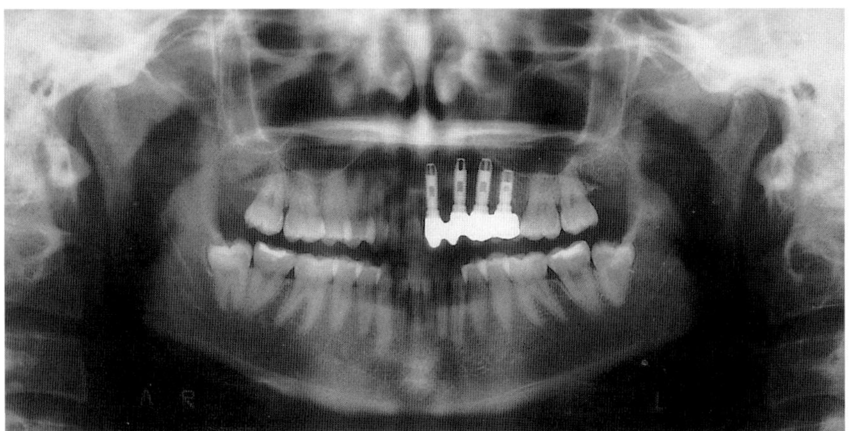
Fig. C7.6

TREATMENT CARRIED OUT

1. Surgical stage 1: four (Branemark) implants (3 × 17 mm and 1 × 10 mm in length with standard 4 mm diameter fixtures inserted). (Fig. C7.3). Patient's RPD modified to serve as a transitional denture.
2. Surgical stage 2: implants exposed and Mirus cone abutments placed, owing to limited space available for the prosthesis (Fig. C7.4 mirror view).
3. Fixed–fixed metal ceramic bridge (21–25) inserted (Figs. C7.5, C7.6 and C7.7).

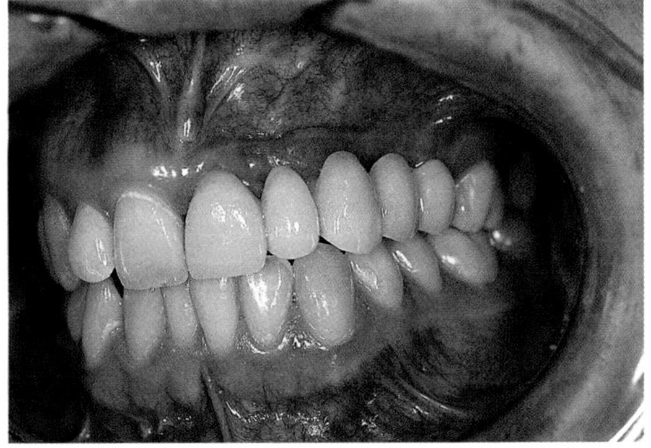
Fig. C7.7

Planning Case 8

Dr I.F. – Age 63 years	
Occupation	Medical practitioner
Complaint	Loss of the bridge replacing the upper right 2nd premolar and 1st molar. Since loss of bridge 1 year ago, the patient has experienced some difficulty in eating.
Past medical history	Heart murmur, but antibiotic cover not needed for dental treatment.
Past dental history	The bridge had been in place for 18 years. 17 failed because of caries. The bridge was sectioned, leaving the crown on 14 and 17 was extracted. Oral hygiene – reasonable (no BPE>1).
Findings	Stable occlusion, with sufficient space between 17,16,15 and 14 and the opposing ridge for implant superstructure. Good bone levels in area of 17,15 but reduced bone level in 16 region. An OPG radiograph revealed that the maxillary antrum was close to the ridge crest in 16 region (Fig. C8.1).
Social history	Non-smoker, keen to maintain a good occlusion.

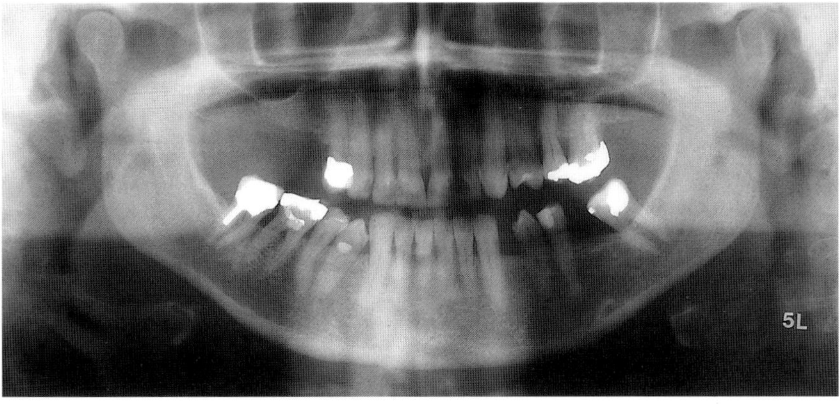

Fig. C8.1

Charting

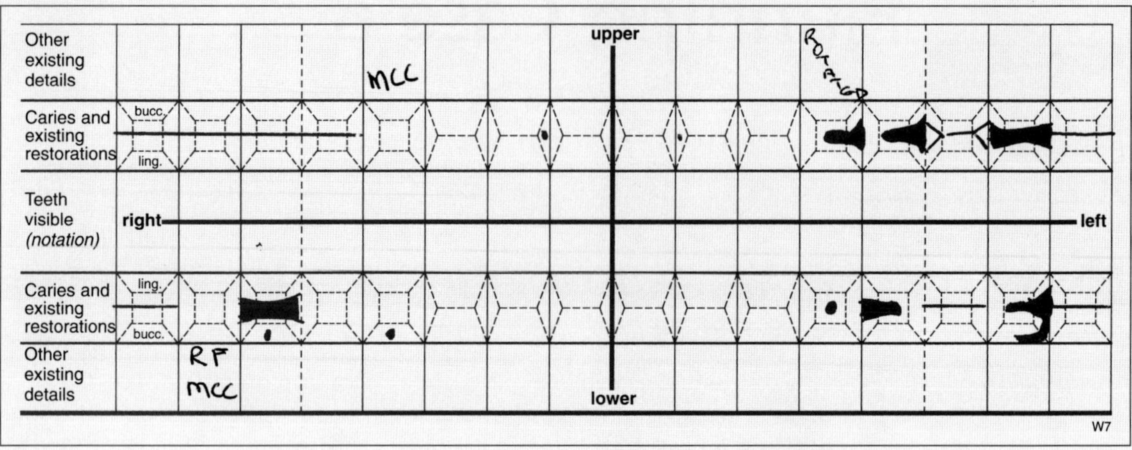

Chart 8.1

TREATMENT OPTIONS

1. Do nothing
2. A removable, metal frame maxillary RPD
3. Cantilever a single unit of bridgework off 14
4. Fixed implant bridge supported on three implants.

Comments

1. Doing nothing is unacceptable, owing to social and functional demands of the patient.
2. RPD: problem of retention and support, and also patient preference against the RPD.
3. Fixed prosthesis: it is unlikely that the functional problems would be addressed by a single unit cantilevered bridge to the upper premolar tooth.

TREATMENT AGREED

1. Provision of fixed implant prosthesis with three standard diameter Nobel Pharma implants. (Two 13 mm implants and one 10 mm implant to avoid the floor of the maxillary antrum were placed at the first surgical visit.)
2. After uncovering of the implants and placement of the abutments (Fig. C8.2 – mirror view), a porcelain fused to metal bridge was screwed on to the tapered EsthetiCone abutments (Fig. C8.3).
3. Because of bone loss in 16 region, this unit had to be constructed with a long clinical crown (Fig. C8.4).
4. The partial fixed implant prosthesis has been in place for 8 years.

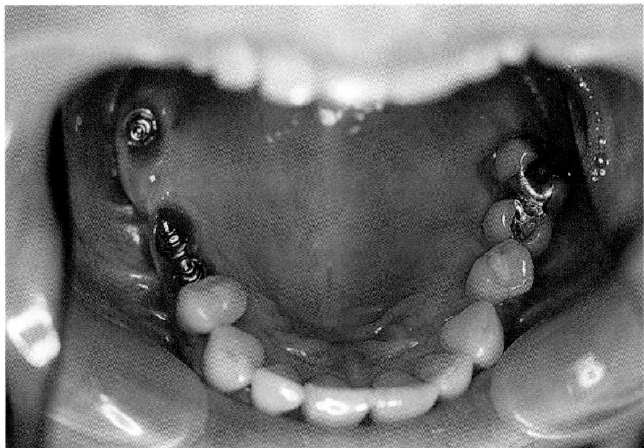

Fig. C8.2 Mirror view.

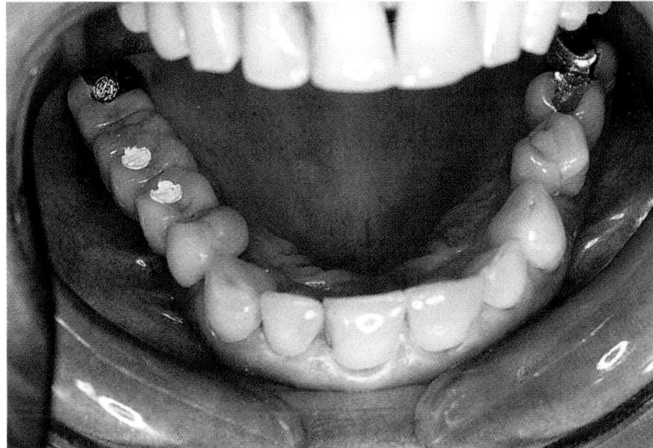

Fig. C8.3 Mirror view.

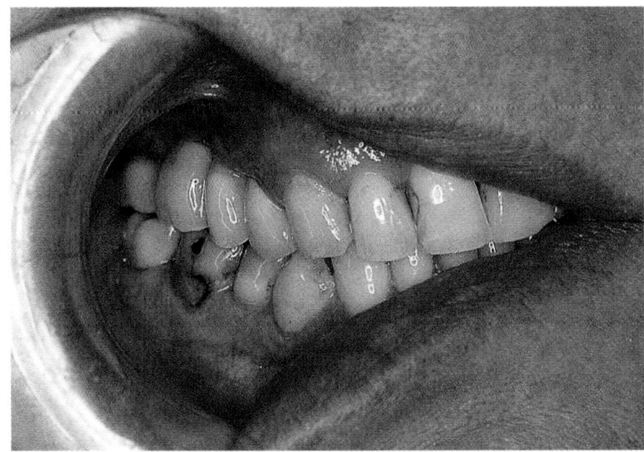

Fig. C8.4

Planning Case 9

Mrs A.M. – Age 67 years	
Occupation	Retired languages teacher
Complaint	Loose lower complete denture.
Past medical history	Nil relevant.
Past dental history	Edentulous for 11 years: lower anterior teeth were the last to be extracted. Never been comfortable with the lower denture – always loose, and speaking French was problematic.
Findings	Mandibular ridge very resorbed posteriorly (Atwood V), relatively prominent in the anterior region but ridge narrow in this region (Atwood IV) (Figs. C9.1. and C9.2). Atwood III maxillary ridge with domed palate (Fig. C9.3). No problems with the upper denture.
Social history	Non-smoker. Active Francophile and is concerned that her unstable mandibular denture compromises her social activities.
Charting	Edentulous.

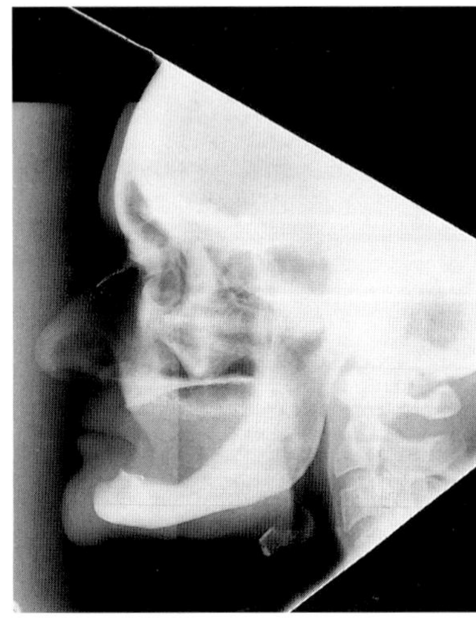

Fig. C9.1

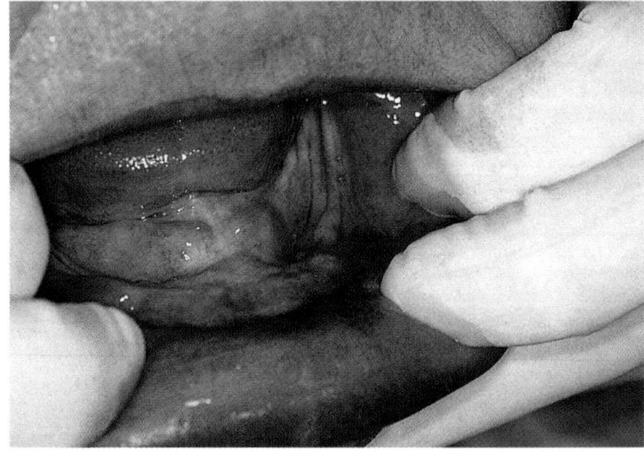

Fig. C9.2

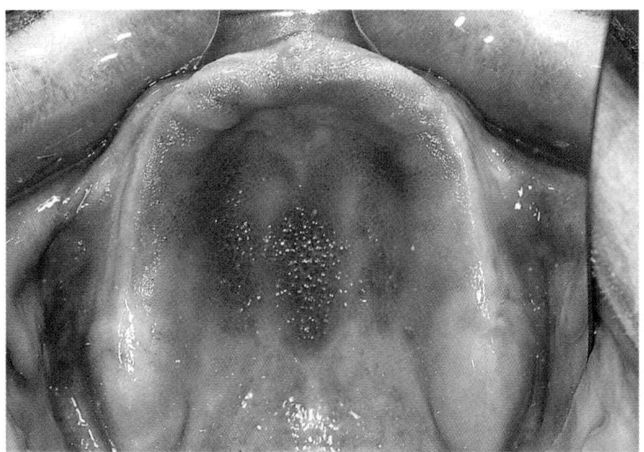

Fig. C9.3 The denture stomatitis was treated by tissue conditioning and antifungal therapy.

TREATMENT OPTIONS

1. Relining current dentures
2. Conventional complete dentures
3. A conventional complete upper denture and an implant-stabilized lower overdenture utilizing two implants placed in the region of the canines
4. A conventional upper complete denture and a fixed bridge supported by five implants in the lower anterior region between the mental foramina
5. Implant-supported/retained overdentures in maxillary and mandibular arches
6. Implant-supported fixed bridges in the maxillary and mandibular arches.

Comments

1. The option of relining the dentures might apply if minimal ridge resorption had occurred and the state of the upper and lower dentures was good.
2. Conventional complete dentures: a lower denture has in the past proved to be problematic. This option, and indeed the option of a copy technique, is unlikely to be successful.
3. The option of a complete upper denture opposed by an implant-supported mandibular overdenture is an attractive simple solution.
4. A more complex option is a conventional complete upper denture opposed by an implant-supported bridge. This option, however, does carry the very real problems of accelerated residual ridge resorption in the maxilla, and should only be considered if the maxilla has an optimal denture-bearing area proved to be stable for many years.
5. If not, then a maxillary implant-supported prosthesis might be sensible.

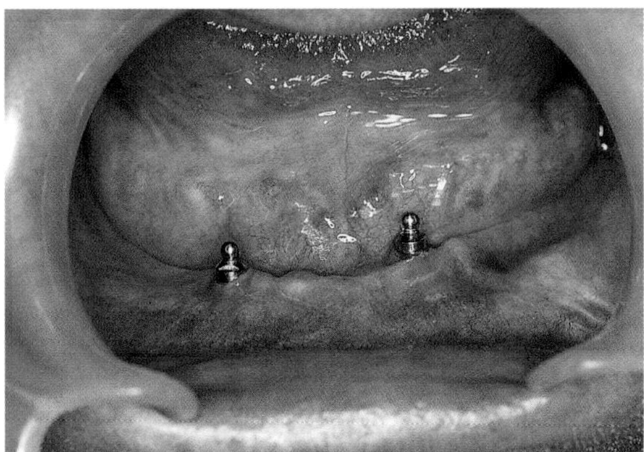

Fig. C9.4

TREATMENT AGREED

1. Because of the need to replace lost alveolar bone as well as the missing teeth, it was decided to utilize the overdenture option. Also, there was the concern that a fixed restoration in the lower jaw would adversely effect the stability of the upper denture.
2. At the first surgical stage, two 15 mm long Astra Tech implants were placed in the canine region.
3. After osseointegration, the fixtures were uncovered and ball attachments were used for retention of the complete mandibular denture (Figs. C9.4 and C9.5).
4. The implants have been in place for 10 years. The dentures were remade after 6 years because of overclosure, owing to wear of the artificial teeth and looseness of the upper denture (Fig. C9.6).

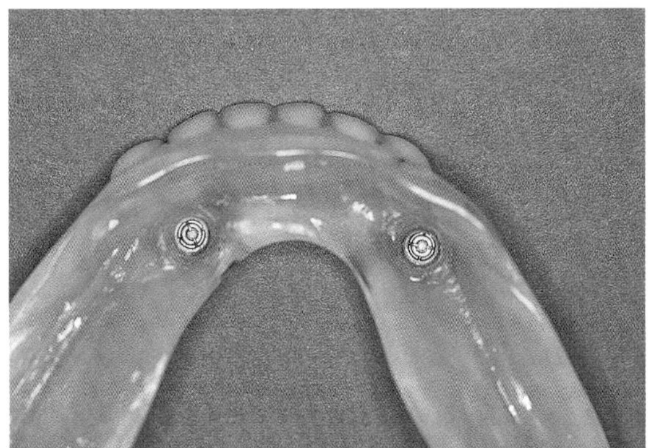

Fig. C9.5

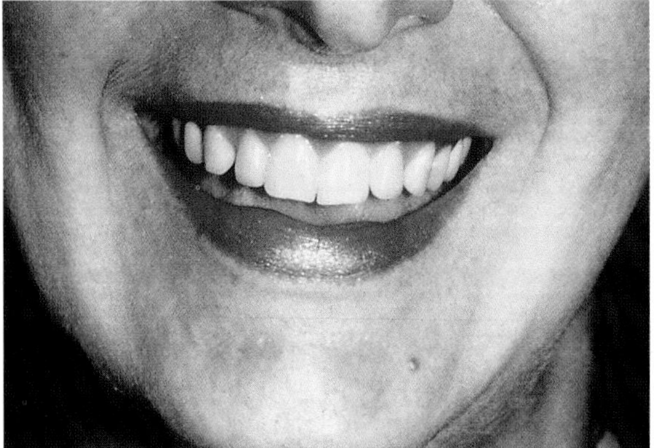

Fig. C9.6

Planning Case 10

Mr J.T. – Age 28 years	
Occupation	Student
Complaint	Problems of eating and, increasingly, of appearance.
Past medical history	Type I ectodermal dysplasia.
Past dental history	Regular attender, as patient is concerned about his dentition. This patient has moderate hypodontia (oligodontia).
Findings	Had received cosmetic improvement of maxillary arch with composite additions (COMP) to crowns of 34,53, 52, 62,63 and 64. Short small deciduous mandibular teeth not evident below lower lip in speech/smiling. Radiograph indicates very short roots in mandibular teeth (Fig. C10.1). Good mandibular bone height and density, and good root formation for 17,16,11,21,65,37,36 and 47 Short roots on 54 and 64.
Social history	Nil relevant.

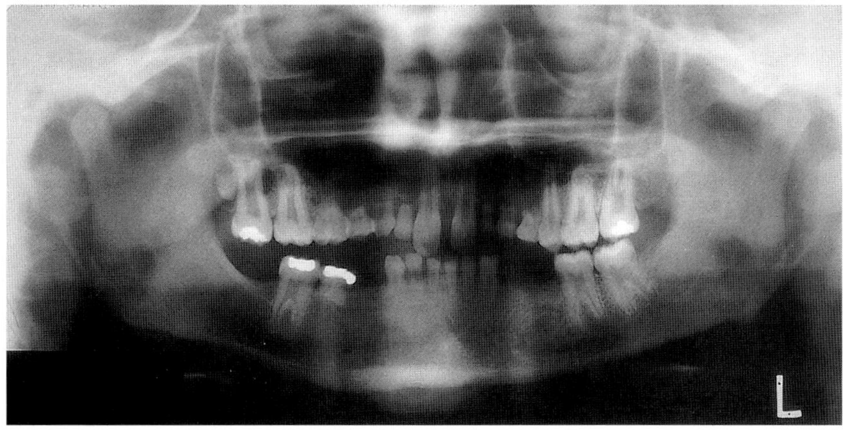

Fig. C10.1

Charting

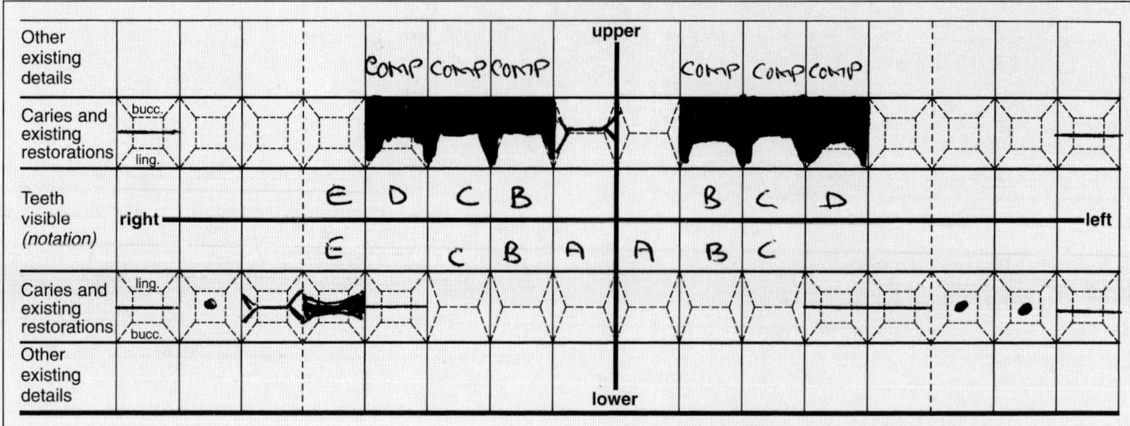

Chart 10.1

TREATMENT OPTIONS

1. Extract deciduous mandibular teeth and provide immediate -/P with Adam's cribs (doing nothing cannot be an option here, nor is rendering edentulous!)
2. Renew RPD with metal frame
3. Restore with a hybrid prosthesis (i.e. fixed component and removable component)
4. Replace transitional partial denture with fixed implant prosthesis using 5/6 implants.

Comment

1. Doing nothing may be appropriate in younger patients, but progressive root resorption of the deciduous teeth heralds the imminent loss of the mandibular deciduous teeth.
2. The immediate mandibular RPD is only a short-term option.
3. The natural form of the secondary dentition affords minimal support retention and stability for any RPD.
4. It is feasible that a hybrid prosthesis could be made using telescopic crowns on the mandibular molars.
5. This is a sensible option which preserves the permanent mandibular teeth and restores function and aesthetics.

TREATMENT CARRIED OUT

1. Extraction of mandibular deciduous teeth and provision of a transitional prosthesis.
2. Surgical stage 1: five implants 3.75 mm in diameter inserted (2 × 10 mm in length and 3 × 15 mm in length). Transitional RPD modified.
3. Surgical stage 2: implant fixtures exposed and abutments placed (Fig. C10.2).
4. Fixed bridge placed to restore the mandibular arch (Figs. C10.3, C10.4).
5. Return to GDP for maintenance and monitoring.

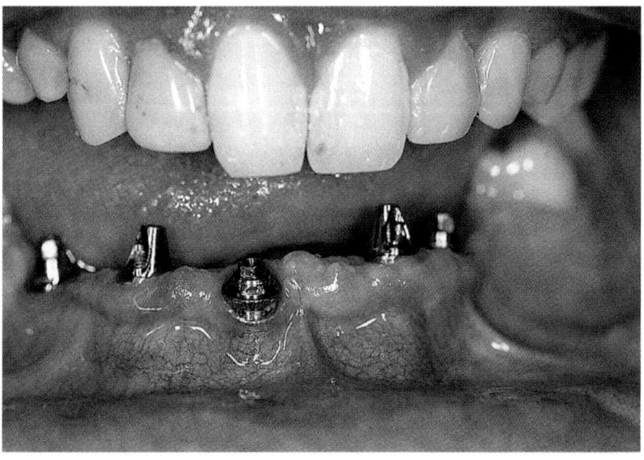

Fig. C10.2

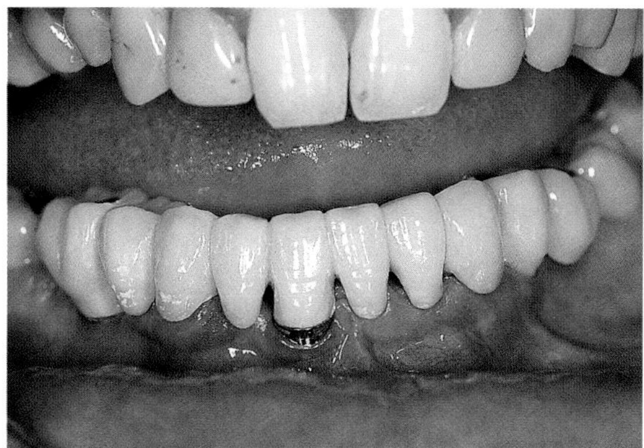
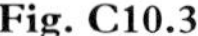
Fig. C10.3

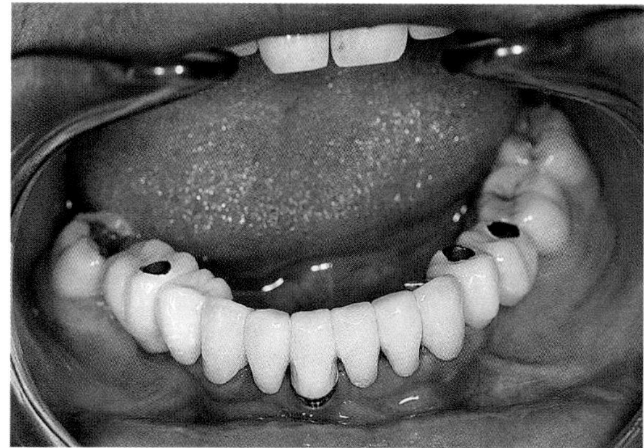
Fig. C10.4

Planning Case 11

Mr N.S. – Age 75 years	
Occupation	Retired engineer
Complaint	Referred by GDP for treatment following loss of a failed bridge in one arch.
Past medical history	Allergic to aspirin, caffeine, penicillin. Inguinal hernia and prostate problems.
Past dental history	Regular dental attender. Had extensive fixed restorations placed over a period of 20 years.
Findings	Well restored with bridgework and crown work, maintained for many years by his GDP. Recent failure of maxillary bridges and previously left mandibular fixed bridge (Fig. C11.1). Right mandibular mesial abutment dubious. Dentist was originally considering restoring the maxilla with crown and bridgework, but now seeks advice, with a request to hand over treatment, on restoring both arches. NB: Patient not keen to leave spans unrestored, nor to have removable prosthesis.

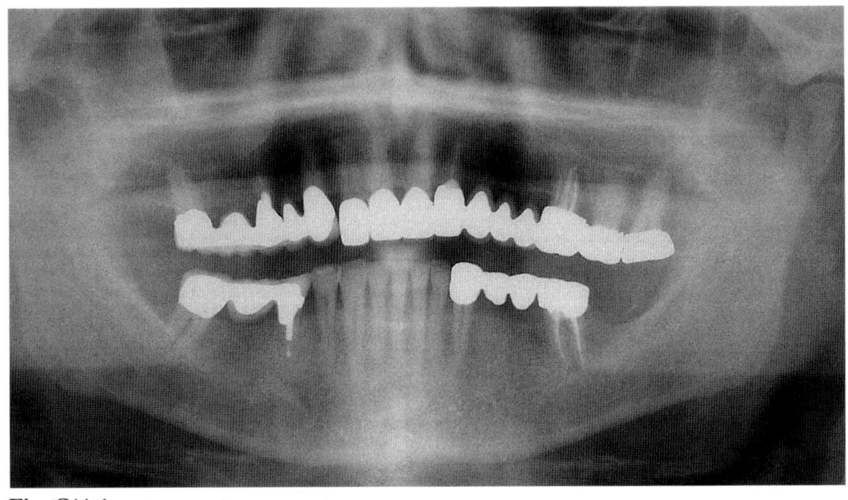

Fig. C11.1

Charting

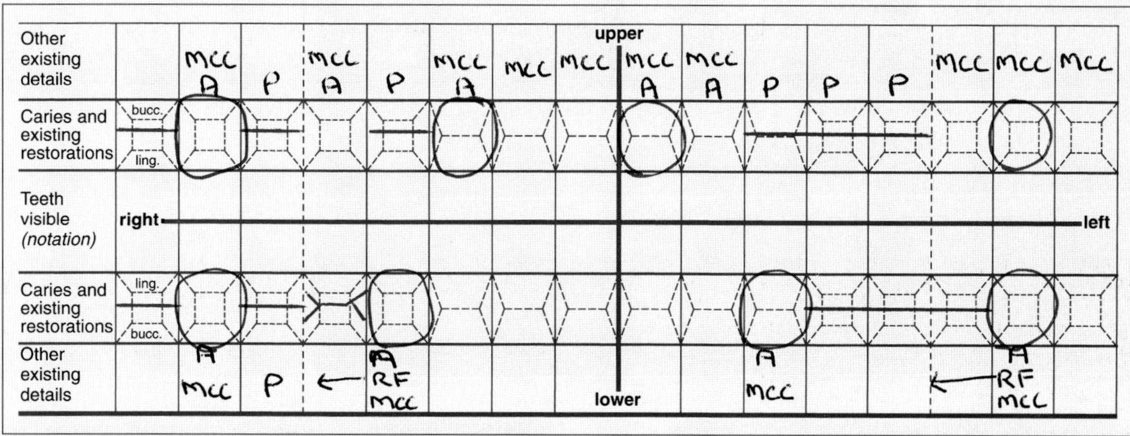

Chart 11.1

Social history Keen socialite, likes dining out.

TREATMENT OPTIONS

1. Do nothing
2. Dismantle bridges, monitor and reassess
3. Restore with RPD in maxilla only and remove failed bridge components
4. Restore U/L arches with RPDs
5. Place maxillary implants, restore with partial fixed prosthesis
6. Place maxillary and mandibular implants and restore with fixed prostheses.

Comments

1. Doing nothing is clearly not an option.
2. Long-term stability of any maxillary RPD is problematic, and the patient would prefer not to have a removable option. Moreover, in this instance full arch occlusal contact would be lost.
3. Two other issues are that the maxillary RPD might have a deleterious affect on remaining fixed components, and failure to restore the lower arch would not satisfy the patient's request to return to comfortable occlusal function.
4. See above.
5. The option of conventional mandibular bridgework would only extend the arch by one unit on the left side and would risk the abutment teeth on the right side. This does not address the problem of the lower arch.
6. The placement of maxillary and mandibular implants and subsequent restoration of the arches with fixed protheses was most acceptable to the patient, and also the one that might have the most durable outcome, although continuous monitoring would be required!

TREATMENT CARRIED OUT

1. Removal of failed bridges in all four quadrants and the provision of an upper RPD as a transitional prosthesis. In addition, the following teeth were extracted: 27, 37 and 45. Endodontic therapy was carried out on 21, 33 and 47.
2. Maxillary RPD provided as a transitional prosthesis over the review/monitoring period. (Patient objected to the presence of 'spaces' and to wearing maxillary RPD.
3. Surgery stage 1: three implants placed in the left maxilla (23,24 and 26 regions) and six placed in the mandible in the positions equating to 37,36,34, and three in the right

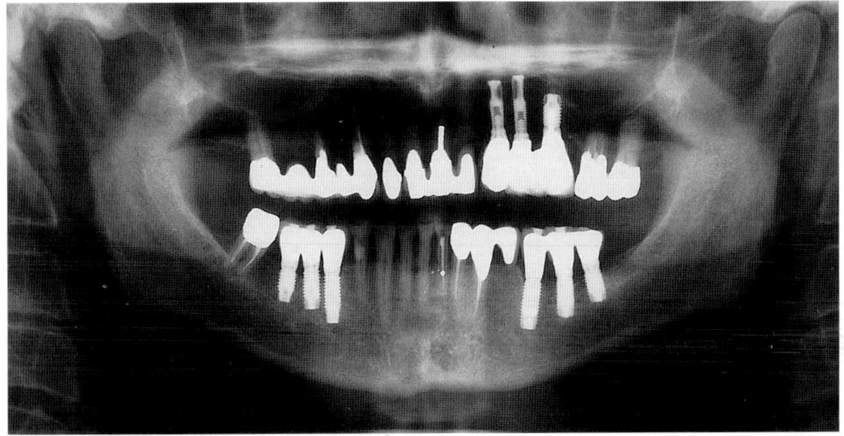
Fig. C11.2

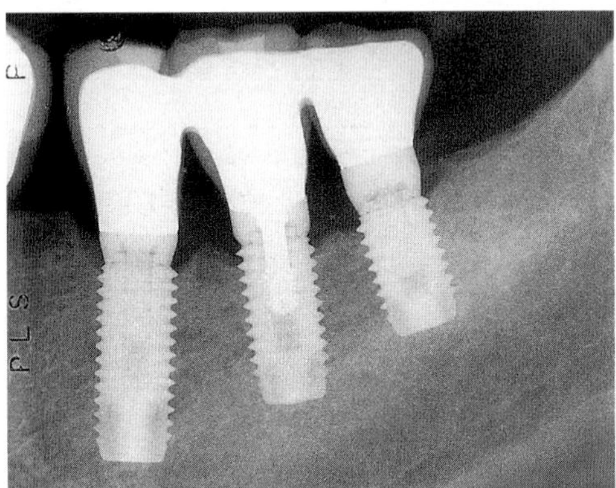

Fig. C11.3

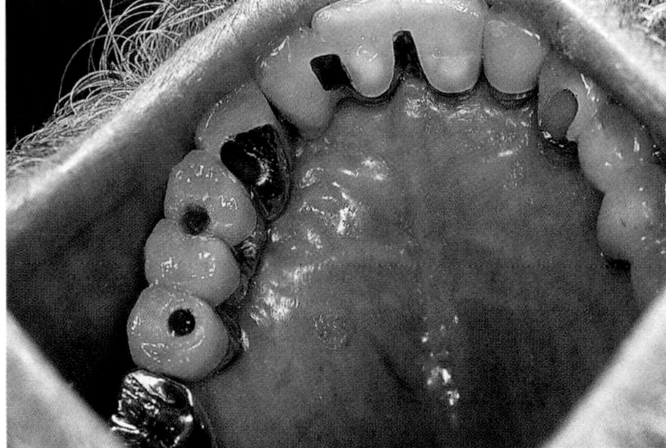
Fig. C11.5 Mirror view.

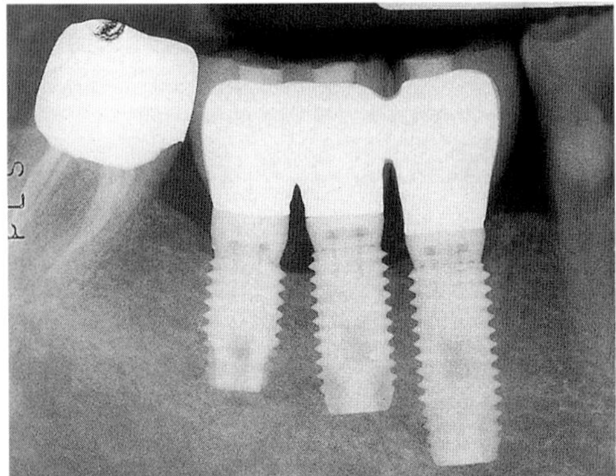

Fig. C11.4

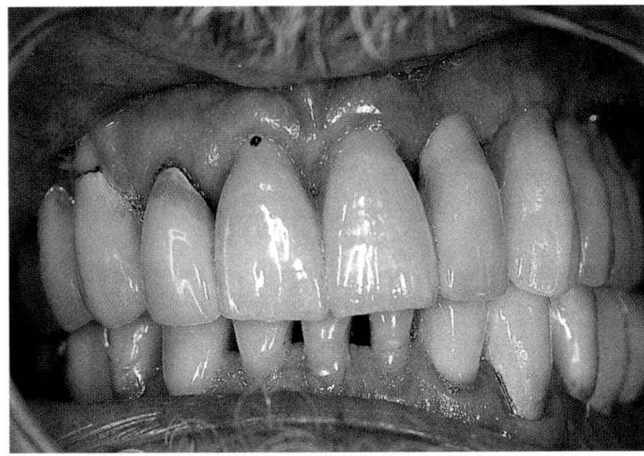
Fig. C11.6

mandibular span between 44 and 47 (Figs C11.2, C11.3 and C11.4).

4. Five months later, and after the second surgical stage, the restorative phase commenced.
5. The lower fixed prostheses were placed.
6. The maxillary fixed prosthesis was placed (Figs C11.5 (mirror view) and C11.6).

Planning Case 12

Mrs S.C. – Age 43 years	
Occupation	Teacher
Complaint	Lost tooth previously anchoring fixed–movable bridge, upper left quadrant. Now very unhappy with her appearance and is experiencing difficulty chewing efficiently.
Past medical history	Nil relevant.
Past dental history	Regular attender, had two fixed–movable bridges placed 15 years ago in each upper quadrant to replace missing premolars (15 and 24, 25), lost owing to failed large restorations. Upper left quadrant bridge failed and extracted 2 years ago following bad taste from 26. Gross caries diagnosed and 26 extracted.
Findings	Moderately heavily restored mouth, no active caries. 23 post-and-core retained porcelain-bonded crown with distal matrix in situ. Bridge in upper left quadrant functioning well, aesthetically good. Occlusion well intercuspated. Group function left lateral excursion, canine guided on right. No BPE >1. Good ridge form (Figs C12.1, C12.2, C12.3 and C12.4). Lack of thickness of maxillary bone overlying antrum. No periapical pathology. No utilizable undercuts on maxillary posterior teeth.

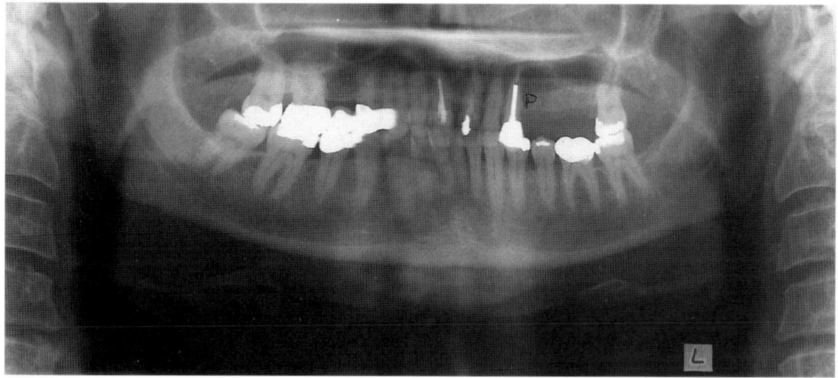

Fig. C12.1

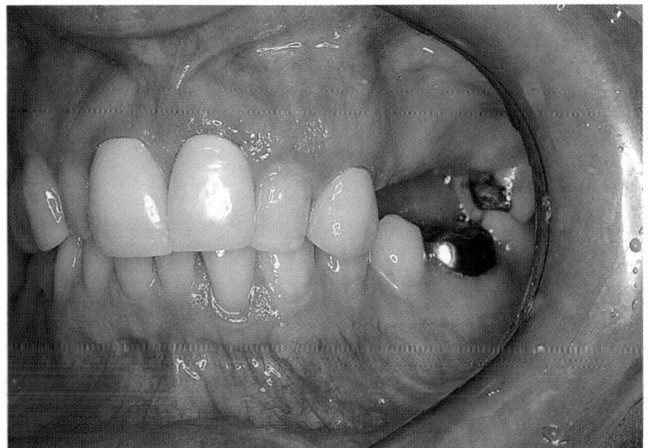

Fig. C12.2

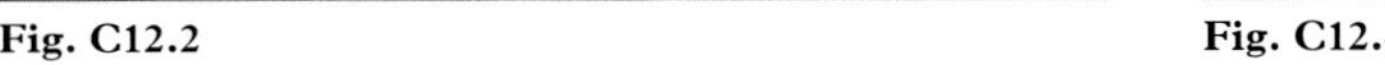

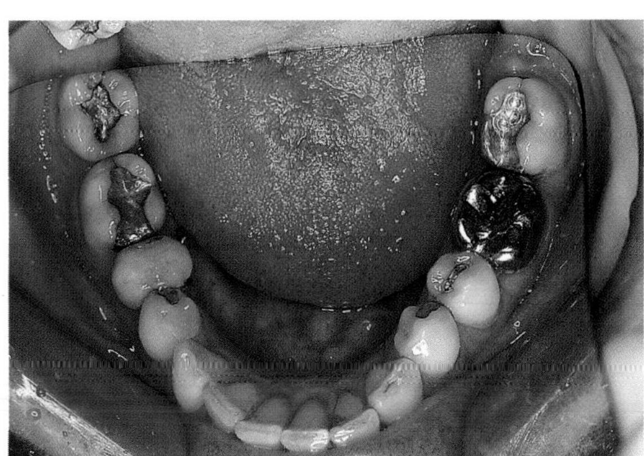

Fig. C12.4

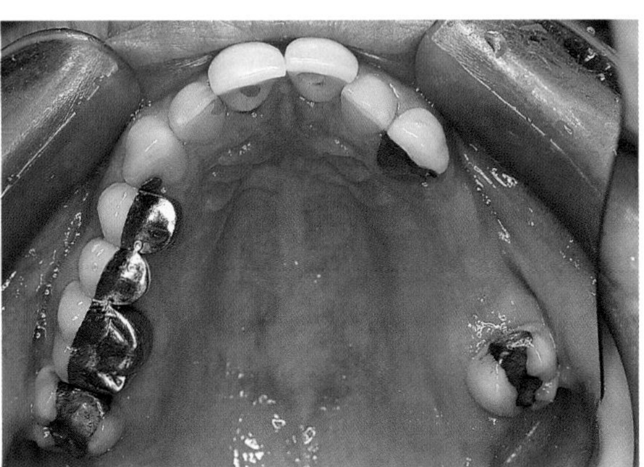

Fig. C12.3

Charting

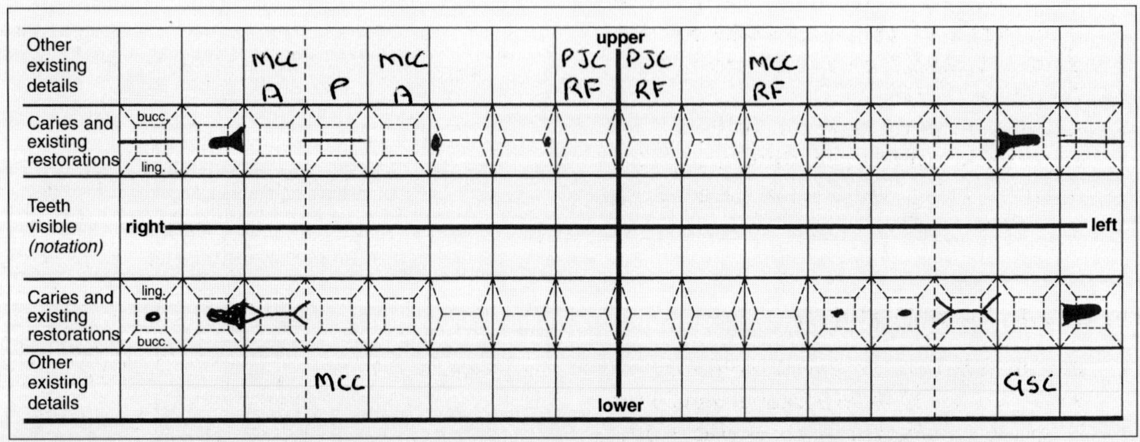

Chart 12.1

Social history

Non-smoker.

TREATMENT OPTIONS

1. Do nothing
2. Construct maxillary RPD
3. Section bridgework, remove 14 pontic, replace 13, 16 crowns, replace 23 crown and crown 27, and provide a metal framed, tooth-supported P/- with appropriate cross-arch bracing
4. Perform a sinus lift and augment the maxillary ridge before placing a single implant and constructing an implant-retained single-tooth prosthesis replacing premolars
5. Provide a fixed–fixed bridge 23–27
6. Crown 23, 27 and provide a precision-retained unilateral RPD.

Comments

1. Doing nothing is not a realistic option here, nor is rendering the patient edentulous.
2. Patient very reluctant to have full palatal coverage. Potential difficulties in producing a satisfactorily stable denture.
3. A lot of treatment, including removal of a satisfactory prosthesis. It is recommended that in such instances the clinician and his/her technician are fully aware of the importance of integrating this form of treatment.
4. Considerable operative intervention required and the patient is unprepared to undergo treatment under a general anaesthetic.
5. Very long span, short clinical crowns and a minor retainer (post on 23) – bridgework contraindicated. The comments for option 2 are relevant here.
6. Just sufficient clinical crown height to accommodate precision attachments. This option would act as a stress-breaker for the post crown in 23.

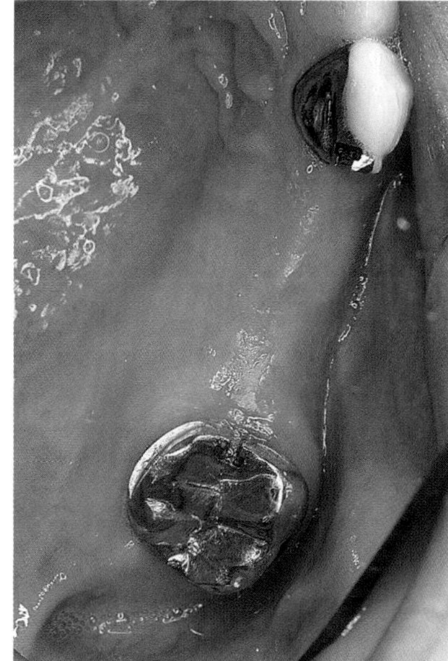

Fig. C12.5

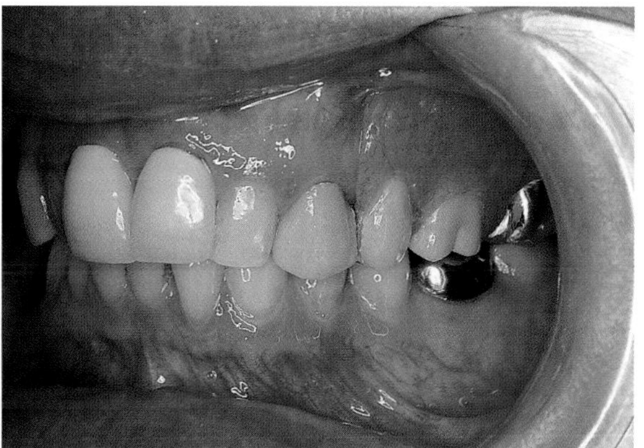

Fig. C12.6

TREATMENT CARRIED OUT

1. Porcelain-bonded crown 23, gold full veneer crown 27 incorporating McCollum precision attachment matrices (Fig. C12.5).
2. A unilateral RPD with metal substructure holding McCollum patrices (Figs C12.6 and C12.7).

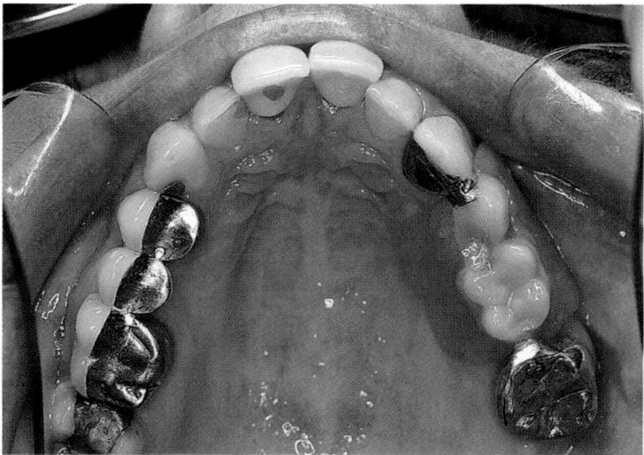

Fig. C12.7

Planning Case 13

Mr P.R. – Age 22 years	
Occupation	Student
Complaint	Concerned about wear on anterior teeth. Has noticed this worsening over last year. Has difficulty chewing any foods and has some TMJ pain on left side.
Past medical history	Nil relevant.
Past dental history	Had two bridges placed posteriorly when 17 years old to replace missing lower premolars lost for orthodontic purposes and first molars lost in childhood due to caries. Orthodontic treatment left spaces in lower arch, and bridges then placed. Aware of clenching teeth when stressed.
Findings	Marked skeletal III facial profile. Occlusion: posterior open bite (Figs C13.1., C13.2 and C13.3). Sole occlusal contact 22 with 33. 22 exhibiting sign of occlusal wear. Occlusal clearance between 17, 48 and 27, 38 about 1 mm. RCP=ICP. No major lateral components during chewing. No BPE >1, however long connectors on lower bridges, leading to localized plaque accumulation and gingival irritation. No periapical pathology. Mounted on semiadjustable articulator. Diagnostic wax-up shows large increase in clinical crown height necessary to make posterior contact on left side.

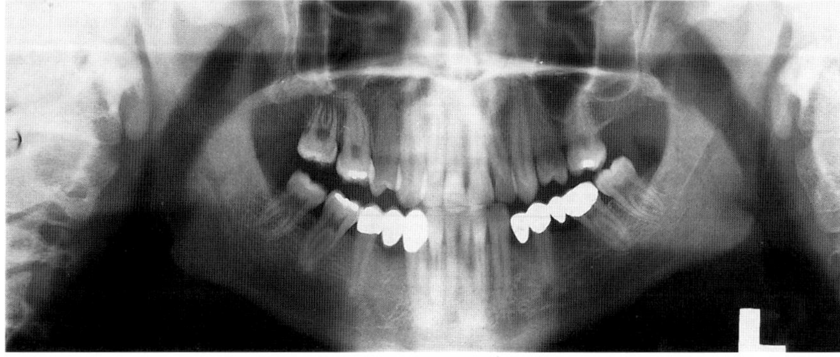

Fig. C13.1

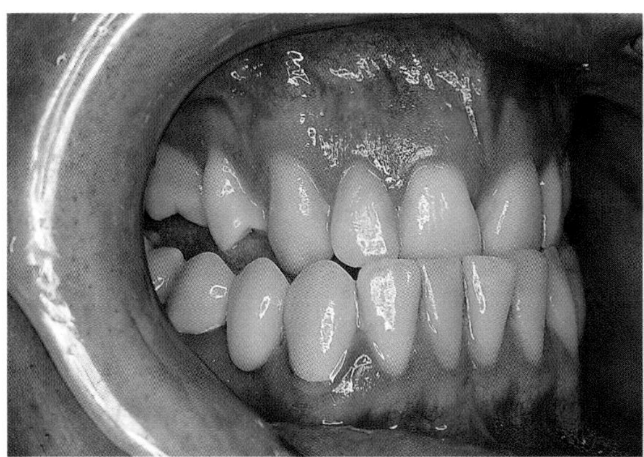

Fig. C13.2

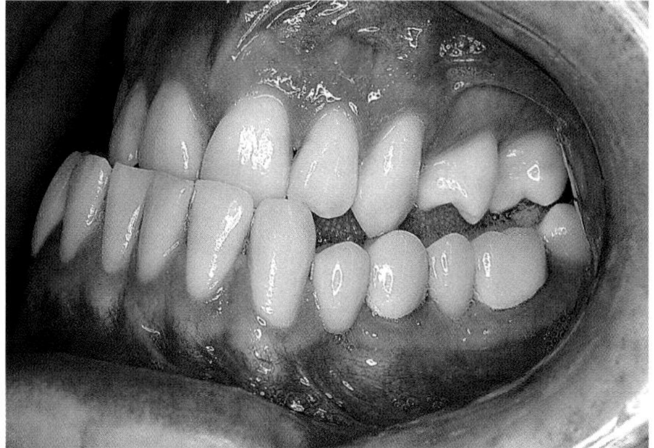

Fig. C13.3

TREATMENT OPTIONS

1. Do nothing, but monitor tooth wear
2. Long-term occlusal splint therapy
3. Liaison with orthodontics re ?orthognathic surgery
4. Replacement of bridgework left and right sides.

Comments

1. As toothwear has increased recently (according to patient) and more would have to occur to allow the posterior natural teeth to come into contact, this is not a reasonable option.
2. This may help reduce toothwear and deal with the TMJ problem, but does not really address the issue of the currently 'functionless' bridgework in the lower jaw.
3. The patient was not willing to undergo this treatment following discussion with orthodontists and oral maxillofacial surgeons.
4. The clinical crowns will be very long if function is restored – this may produce an unfavourable crown : root ratio and will place cement lutes under significant shearing forces. Short preparations and a high occlusal plane (Fig C13.4).

Charting

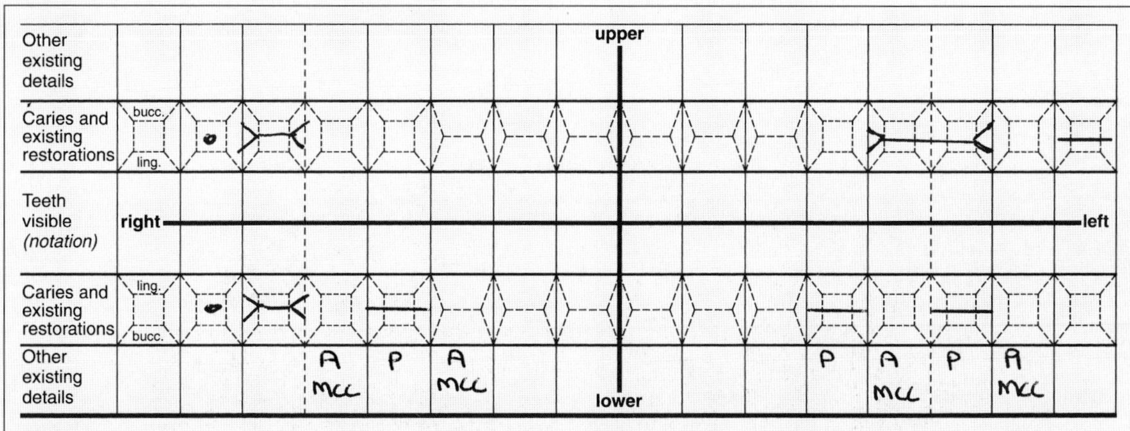

Chart 13.1

Social history	Non-smoker, occasional drinker.

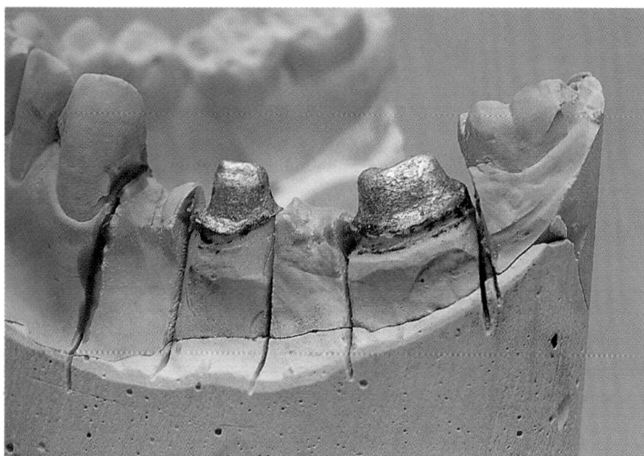

Fig. C13.4

TREATMENT AGREED

1. Composite added to existing bridgework to raise them into function – assess effect on TMJ – if favourable.
2. Laboratory-milled telescopic crowns definitively cemented 35 & 37 using zinc phosphate cement (Fig. C13.5).
3. Provision of compound bridge superstructure (34,35,36,37) cemented using TempBond, restoring occlusal contacts as previously defined by composite (Figs. C13.6. and C13.7.). Any displacing forces will lead to loosening of the bridge, but the telescopic crowns will remain cemented to the abutment teeth (with the stronger cement), protecting them from caries.
4. Fixed–fixed bridge replaced on right side (patient's left) with light occlusal contacts (Fig C13.8).

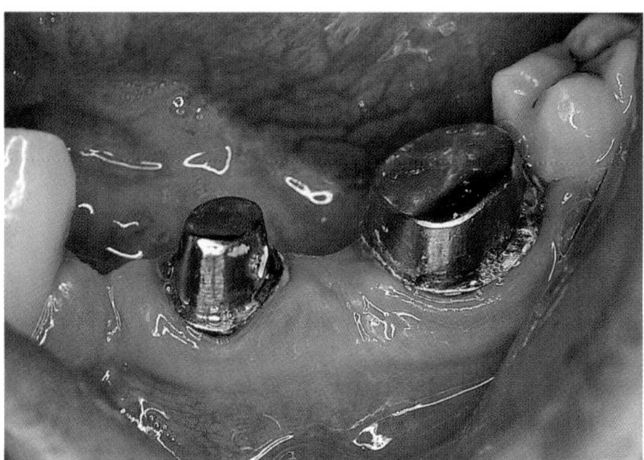

Fig. C13.5

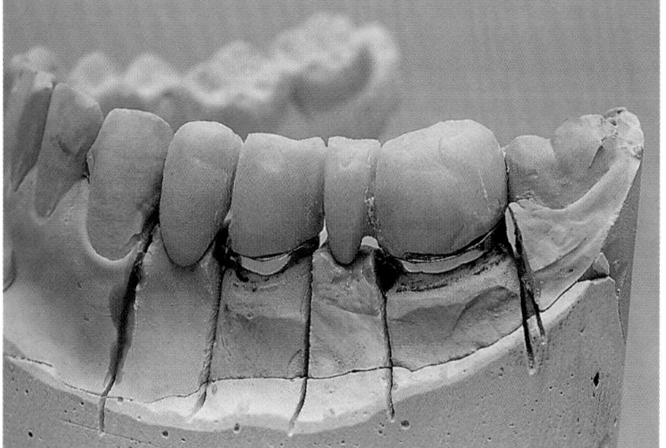

Fig. C13.6

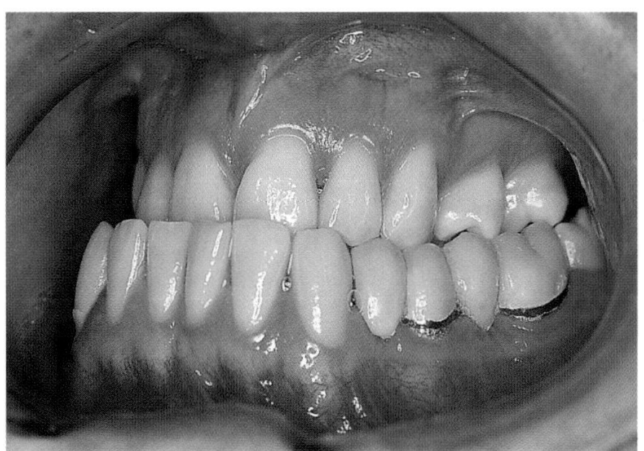

Fig. C13.7

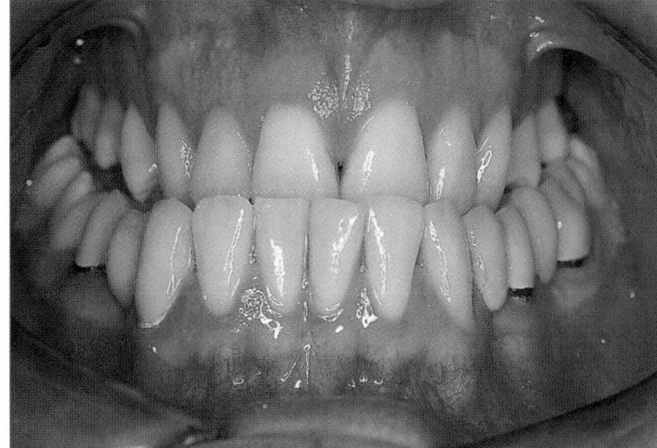

Fig. C13.8

Planning Case 14

Mrs M.E. – Age 40 years	
Occupation	Nurse
Complaint	Lost two lower incisor teeth (41, 31, Fig. C14.1). Complains that lower denture is intrusive to her tongue and that it interferes with speech and eating. Concerned by the appearance of the lower incisors because the teeth are obviously different colours (Figs C14.2. and C14.3).

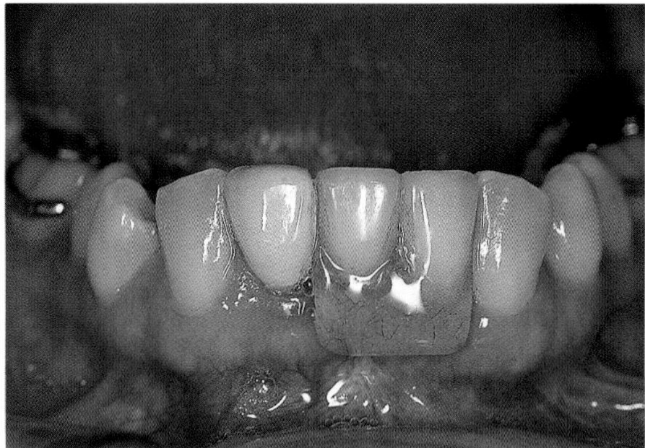

Fig. C14.1

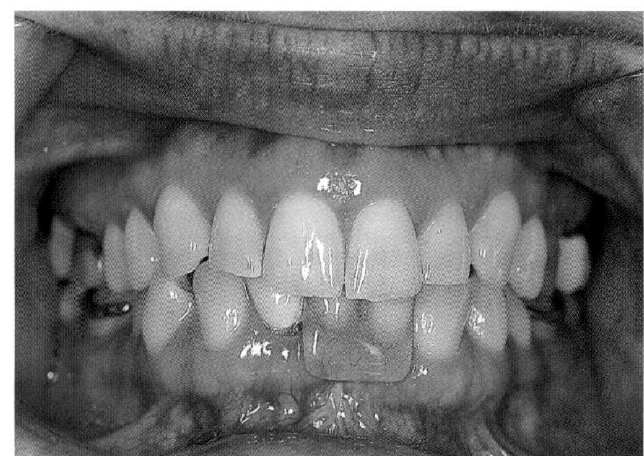

Fig. C14.2

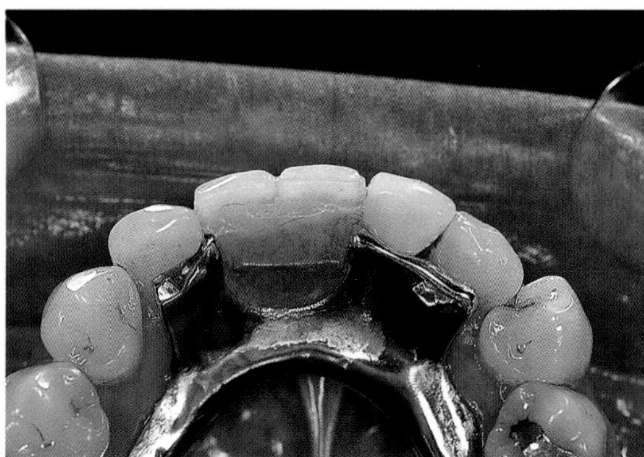

Fig. C14.3

Past medical history	Nil relevant.
Past dental history	Failed endodontic treatment and crowning of lower incisors following childhood trauma. Apical surgery attempted unsuccessfully, otherwise nothing abnormal. All treatment performed under local anaesthesia.
Findings	Moderately restored, well cared-for dentition. Amalgam tattoo in alveolar mucosa below 31. Well intercuspated occlusion with canine guidance on left and right lateral excursions. RCP-ICP slide = 1 mm on bilateral premolar contacts. Tooth-borne mandibular RPD retentive and stable; major connector is a lingual plate, which the patient feels contributes to poor appearance of the prosthesis. PJC on tooth 42. BPE = 0 in all sextants. Good ridge form in edentulous span anteriorly; no other edentulous spaces. No periapical pathology, good root length on abutment teeth. No obvious interference to anterior guidance.

Charting

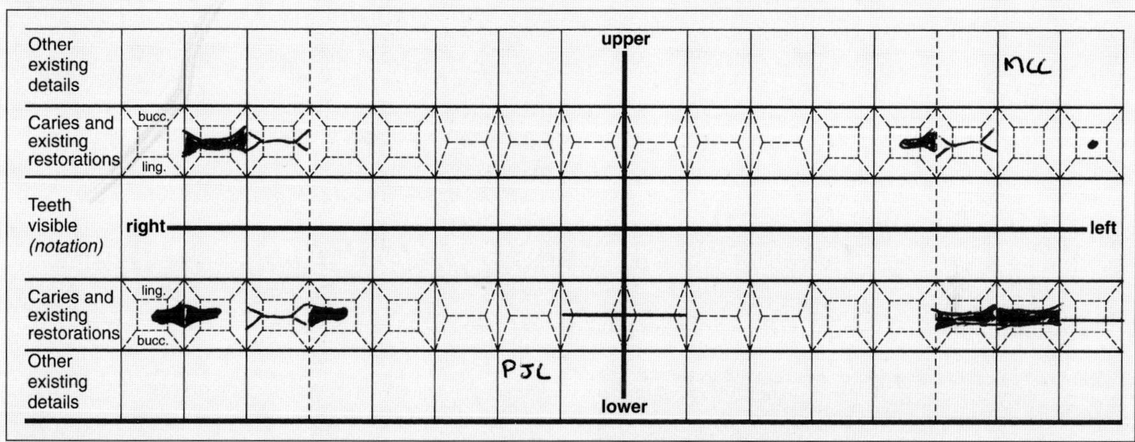

Chart 14.1

Social history	Non-smoker, occasional drinker.

TREATMENT OPTIONS

1. Do nothing, other than primary treatment
2. New RPD with improved extension of the major connector into the lingual. Reduced coverage of lingual plate, better shade selection.
3. Implant-retained crowns replacing missing incisors.
4. Fixed–fixed porcelain-bonded bridge from 42 to 32.
5. Cantilever porcelain-bonded bridge from 42 and cantilever RBB from 32.

Comments

1. Doing nothing to improve the prosthesis is not acceptable to this patient (neither is rendering her edentulous!).
2. There is an increased risk of plaque accumulation with any removable prosthesis that has plate and/or clasp components. The patient was keen to explore less bulky methods of restoration.
3. There is some morbidity associated with this procedure that the patient was not willing to accept.
4. The intact 32 would have to be prepared for a crown. The patient was reluctant to have this performed and wanted as little invasive treatment as possible.
5. As cantilever designs were to be employed, minimal preparation to 32 could be used with a greater probability of success for an RBB.

TREATMENT AGREED

1. Cantilever porcelain-bonded bridge from 42, modifying the existing crown preparation under the existing PJC.
2. Cantilever RBB from 32 (Figs C14.4 and C14.5).
3. The patient's smile was considerably improved by matching tooth/crown shades (Fig. C14.6).

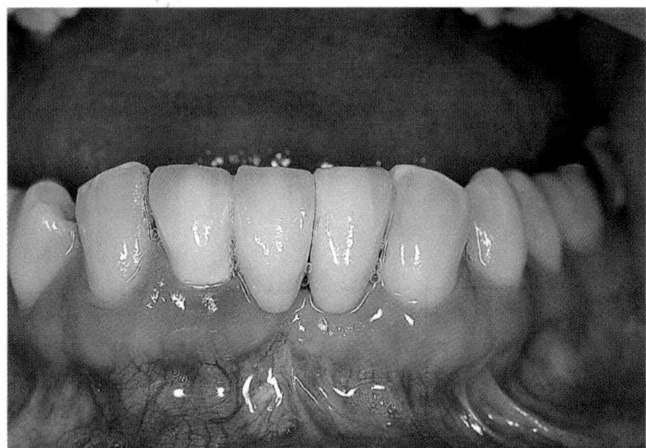

Fig. C14.5

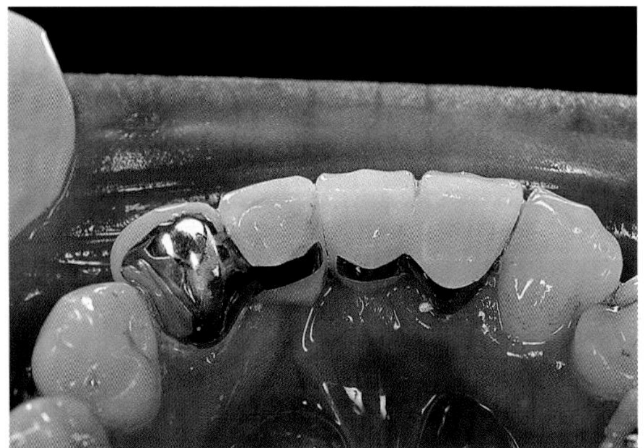

Fig. C14.4

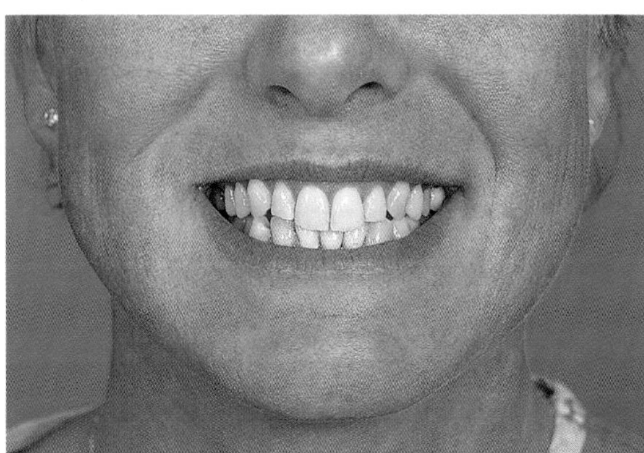

Fig. C14.6

Index

GWENT HEALTHCARE NHS TRUST
LIBRARY
ROYAL GWENT HOSPITAL
NEWPORT